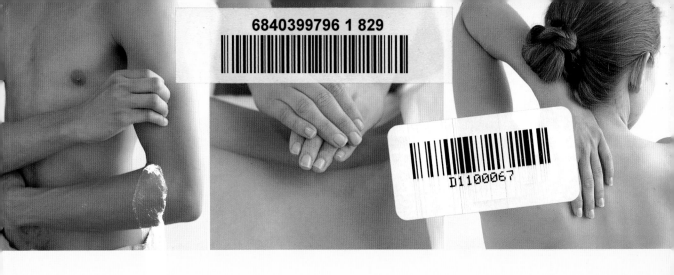

The Body Shop

Massage

Aurum Press

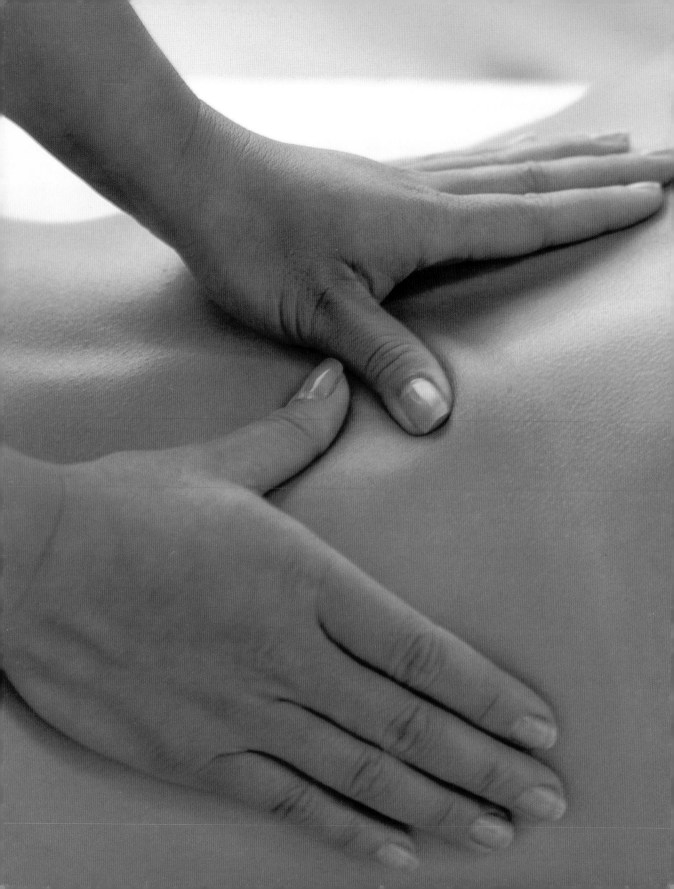

The Body Shop
Massage

monica roseberry

photography by sheri giblin

First Published in Great Britain
2005 by Aurum Press Ltd
25 Bedford Avenue, London WC1B 3AT

THE BODY SHOP INTERNATIONAL, PLC
Founder, Non-Executive Director Dame Anita Roddick
Chairman Adrian Bellamy
Chief Executive Officer Peter Saunders
Director of Product Paul McGreevy
Publications Manager Justine Roddick

WELDON OWEN INC.
Chief Executive Officer John Owen
Chief Operating Officer and President Terry Newell
Vice President and Publisher Roger Shaw
Vice President, International Sales Stuart Laurence

Publisher Rebecca Poole Forée
Creative Director Gaye Allen
Senior Art Director Emma Boys
Art Director Colin Wheatland
Managing Editor Elizabeth Dougherty
Production Director Chris Hemesath
Colour Manager Teri Bell
Co-Edition and Reprint Coordinator Todd Rechner
Designers Rachel Lopez, Adrienne Aquino
Consulting Editor Maria Behan
Anglicization Grant Laing Partnership

The Body Shop Massage was conceived and produced by Weldon Owen Inc.,
814 Montgomery Street, San Francisco, California 94133, United States, in collaboration
with The Body Shop International PLC, Watersmead, Littlehampton, West Sussex,
BN17 6LS, United Kingdom. The Body Shop™ trademark application pending.

A WELDON OWEN PRODUCTION
Copyright © 2005 Weldon Owen Inc.
All rights reserved, including the right of reproduction in whole or in part in any form.

Set in Bembo™ and Benton Gothic™
Colour separations by Bright Arts, Hong Kong
Printed in China by Midas Printing Limited

10 9 8 7 6 5 4 3 2 1
2008 2007 2006 2005

A catalogue record for this book is available from the British Library.

ISBN 1-84513-076-6

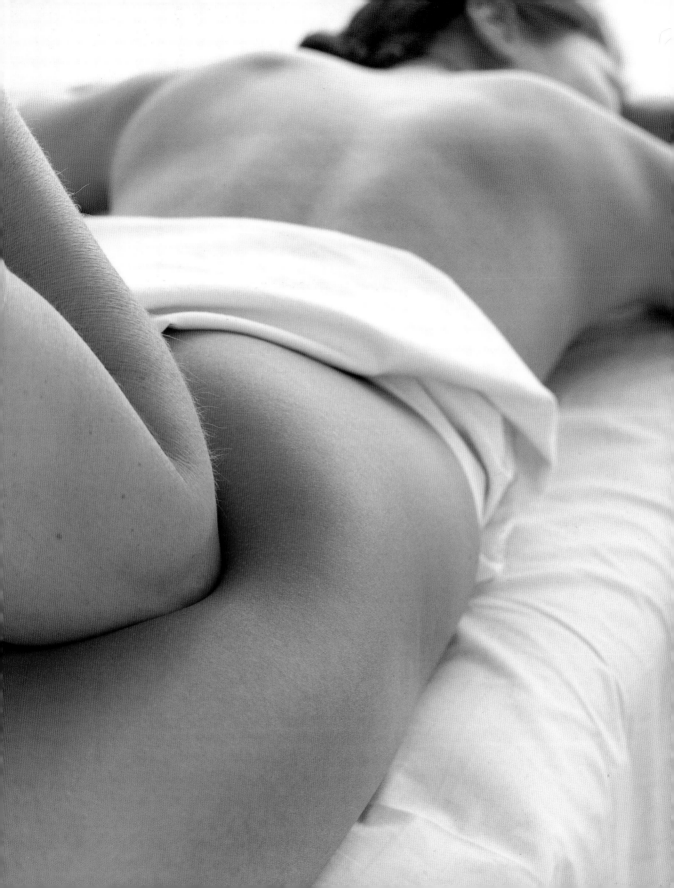

contents

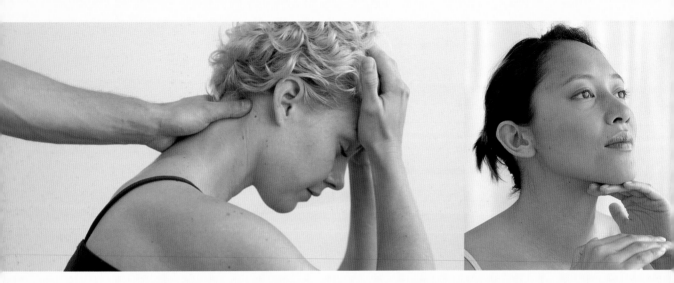

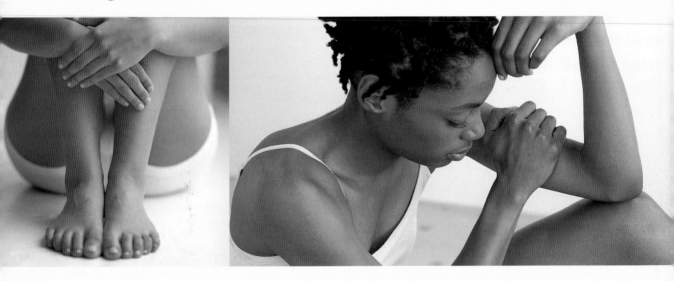

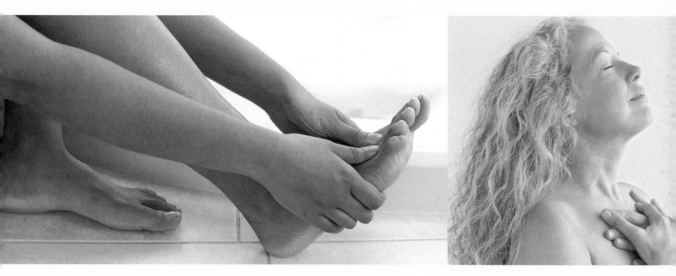

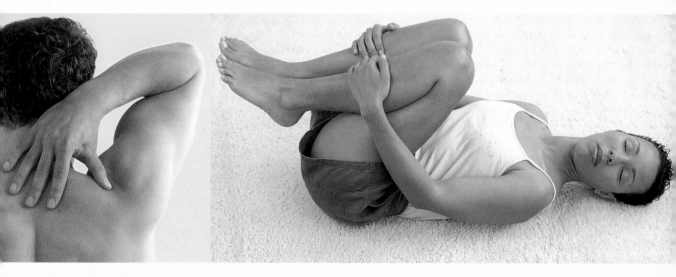

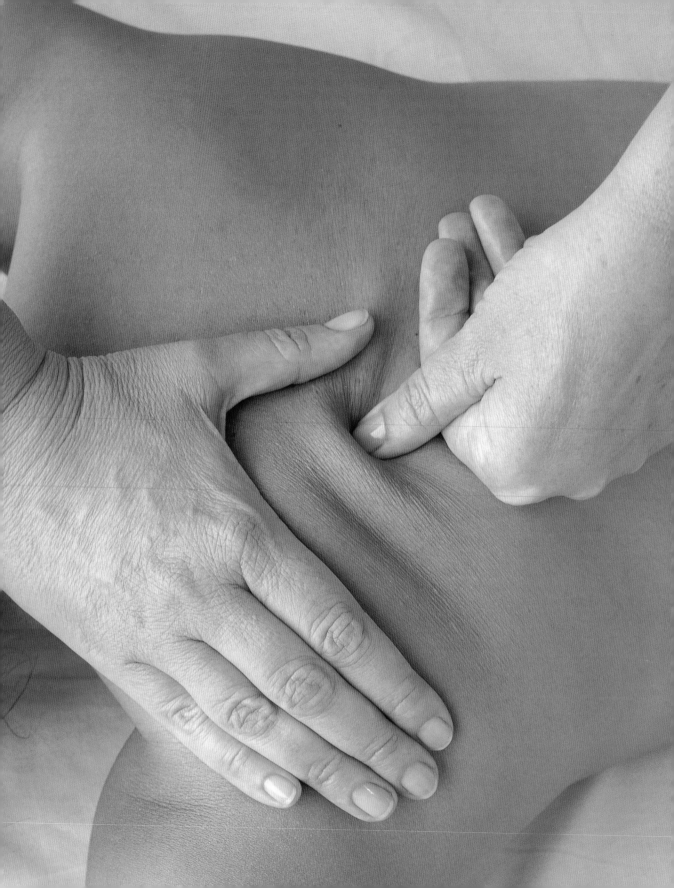

the power of touch

Massage has been practised throughout most cultures for thousands of years for one simple reason: touch is a powerful healer. Today more than ever, as the stress and strain of our fast-paced lives take their toll on our bodies, relationships and enjoyment of life, caring touch is an absolute necessity. Whether it's structured in the form of a massage or just a gentle caress, touch benefits the body, mind and spirit.

Research shows us again and again that touch measurably improves health and wellbeing. According to studies by the Touch Research Institutes, based at the University of Miami, in Florida, touch can facilitate weight gain in premature babies, reduce stress hormones, combat depressive symptoms, alleviate pain and boost the immune system. In dozens of international studies, researchers have found that massage can help reduce anxiety, slow respiratory and heart rates, soothe tension-related headaches and eyestrain, reduce blood pressure, encourage the production of endorphins, and improve alertness at work.

Different forms of healing touch are practised around the globe, from the familiar gliding movements of Swedish massage to the ancient Eastern traditions of acupressure and reflexology. But at the heart of them all are caring touch and a positive intention – whether it's to help relieve pain, to give pleasure or simply to express love.

learning the basics

You don't need to be a massage therapist to give a massage. You can use simple touch techniques to help heal and soothe your friends and loved ones – and even yourself. This book shows you how, drawing on the best massage therapies from around the world. Illustrated step-by-step instructions teach you how to easily weave massage into your daily life, whether at home, work or play, and whether with a partner or on your own.

In many ways, massage is like music: once you know the basic notes, or strokes, you can write a song for any mood, from simple lullabies to elaborate symphonies of sensation. You can ease pain, arouse passion or soothe someone to sleep with a few basic strokes (see pages 14–17 ▶) applied in a variety of ways. And you can give or receive a massage almost anywhere – on sofas, chairs, floors, in the shower, even on an aeroplane. It can be as simple as a five-minute foot rub or as involved as a slow, sensual full-body massage.

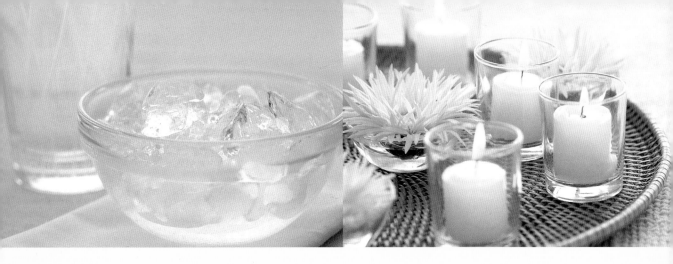

setting the scene

For many treatments, caring hands are all you need to get started. For others, sheets, blankets, pillows, towels, and massage oils, lotions or creams help you make the most of your massage time. Aromatherapy, the use of fragrant essential oils distilled from plants to enhance mood and promote health, can complement the massage experience. For example, lavender oils soothe, while rosemary oils stimulate. (Essential oils should almost never be applied directly to the skin. See page 13 ▸ for information about aromatherapy massage oils.) Some simple massages you can enjoy almost anywhere; for others, a place of calm and comfort greatly enhances the experience. Flickering candles, aromatic oils and soothing music can create a sanctuary far from the cares and stresses of the outside world.

a few notes of caution

Some things to remember: the goal of a massage is for both giver and receiver to feel good, so while working, keep your body relaxed, never use brute force, ask what feels good and stay within your partner's comfort zone. Never apply massage strokes directly on top of the spine or over varicose veins, open wounds, areas of intense pain, skin rashes, infections or bruises. Also do not work on a pregnant woman's abdomen or perform deep massage on her feet or hands. When giving a massage, remember that good posture is vital. Keep your back straight and your head high, and use your leg muscles, not just your hands, to power your strokes. After receiving a massage, especially one with cross-fibre rubbing, drink lots of water to wash away freshly freed toxins. If any area of your body is very sore, apply a cold pack to it for 7–10 minutes before and after massage. For acute or chronic pain, seek professional help. Also see page 13 ▸ for aromatherapy cautions.

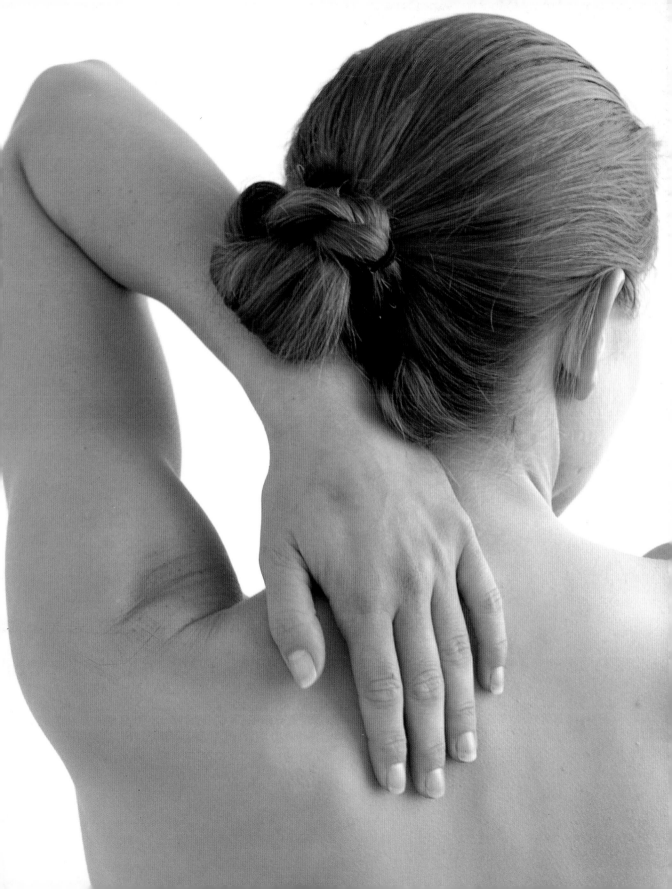

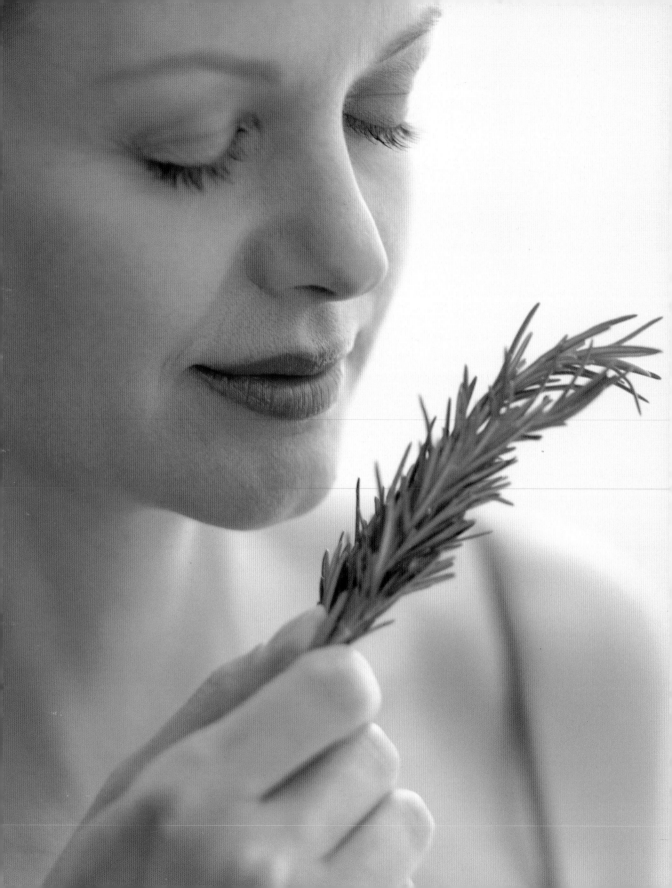

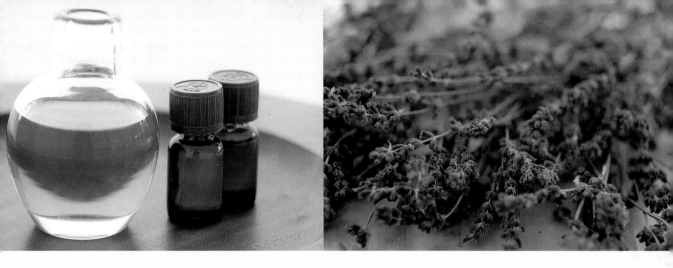

aromatherapy massage oils

You can enhance a massage with aromatherapy essential oils (oils distilled from aromatic plants). The powerful scents and chemical properties of essential oils, such as clary sage, lavender, rosemary, sandalwood and others, have been used for centuries to help ease muscle tension and improve mood. Because essential oils can be extremely potent, they should almost never be applied directly to the skin; first dilute them in an inert oil (called a carrier oil). Always check the amount recommended for the specific oil you're using and stick to the quantities advised. If the person giving or receiving a massage is pregnant or has any serious illnesses or allergies, seek advice from a qualified aromatherapist before using essential oils.

For a more indulgent massage, create your own massage oil by mixing essential oils with a carrier oil, such as grapeseed, sweet almond, sesame or jojoba oil. Different essential oils have different effects. Here are some combinations to try:

Relaxing Massage Oil

50 ml carrier oil

12 drops lavender essential oil

8 drops clary sage essential oil

5 drops ylang-ylang essential oil

Energising Massage Oil

50 ml carrier oil

16 drops geranium essential oil

7 drops rosemary essential oil

2 drops peppermint essential oil

Detoxifying Massage Oil

50 ml carrier oil

8 drops cypress essential oil

8 drops juniper essential oil

5 drops lavender essential oil

4 drops orange essential oil

Sensual Massage Oil

50 ml carrier oil

10 drops patchouli, sandalwood, rose or ylang-ylang essential oil

basic strokes

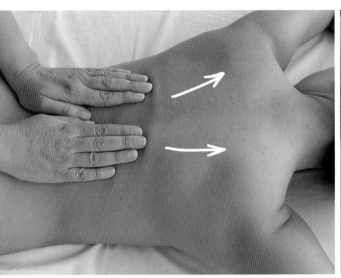

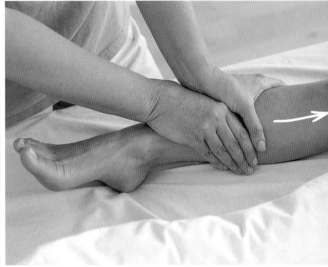

gliding

Gliding strokes are wonderfully relaxing and versatile. For opening strokes, warm some massage oil between your palms and then use light fanning strokes to spread it, so you can glide smoothly and easily. On large areas, such as the back, mould hands to the contours of the body and use long sweeping movements of gradually increasing pressure to cover the entire surface. On smaller surfaces, such as the arms, encircle as much of the limb as possible and lead the stroke with the web of your hand (between the thumb and index finger).

light gliding

For a seamless and flowing massage, use lighter gliding strokes when you start massaging each new area of the body, progress to deeper strokes, and then close with lighter strokes again, skimming over the skin as if you're shaping a perfect sandcastle. Light, gliding strokes can be very calming, while medium pressure eases tight muscles and helps you feel where tension is held, so you can return to the area later to administer deeper strokes.

and pressure of strokes – from short, fast, light strokes to long, slow, deep ones.

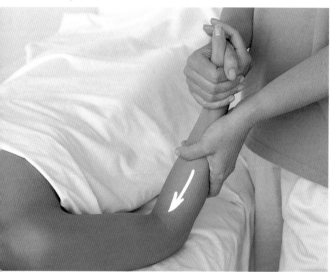 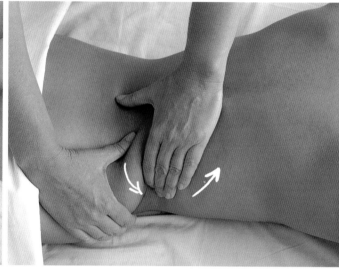

deep gliding

Exercise, stress and even poor diet can leave irritating chemical deposits between muscle fibres, which can cause pain. Flushing those chemicals out creates healthier muscles that respond better and faster and don't wear out as easily. Deep gliding massage strokes create a sweeping effect on the fluids of the body, which helps loosen these deposits.

Deeper gliding also improves circulation, as the strokes help move blood back towards the heart and lungs to load up on oxygen for another trip through the body. Use heavier pressure when stroking towards the heart; lighten up when stroking away from the heart.

kneading

Kneading is a rhythmic movement of rolling and compressing, pushing and pulling, and grasping and releasing muscles to stretch and relax them. Gentle kneading works well on smaller and thinner muscles, while deeper kneading reaches through thicker layers of muscle to loosen stubborn or recurring knots.

When working small muscles, such as those in the shoulders, knead with your thumbs and fingertips, like a cat contently curling her paws. With larger muscles, such as those at the waist, push and pull as if kneading dough. Knead thigh muscles as if wringing a large wet towel.

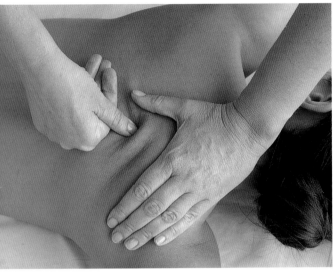
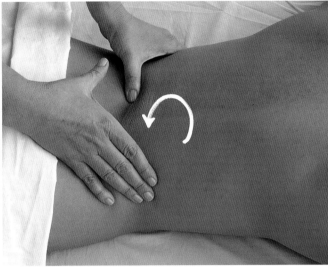

direct pressure

Use localised direct pressure to quell muscle spasms, to activate reflexology points and to stimulate acupressure points. Apply pressure gradually, straight down into the tissue, holding steady with your partner's inhalation and sinking deeper with her exhalation over the course of two or three breaths. The key to using direct pressure is a very slow, incremental release, which causes the muscles to relax more fully afterwards.

circular friction

Sore spots that need extra attention respond well to rapidly repeated motions, including circular friction and thumb-over-thumb pressure. Circular friction can be performed with fingers, thumbs, palms, fists, knuckles, elbows or massage tools. Use pressure deep enough to work into the muscle. Friction circles let you go over a sore spot and come back to it quickly, repeating or building the pressure as you feel the muscles soften.

If your hands tire, use the weight of your body to rock gently, pressing in as you move forwards and releasing as you rock backwards. Using your weight to put pressure behind your movements will help give your hands a break.

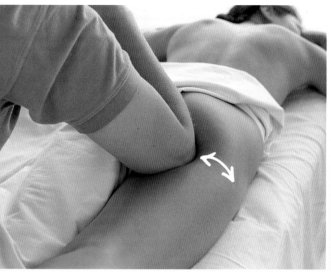

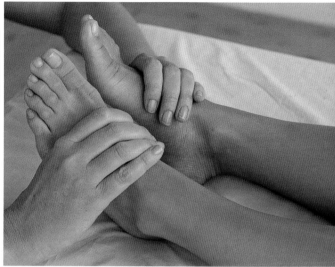

cross-fibre friction

Cross-fibre friction can help to relax tight muscles, especially around old injuries and stubborn knots. Muscle fibres run parallel to each other, sliding against each other thousands of times a day as they relax and contract with every movement. Stress, poor diet, insufficient fluids, poor posture, tiredness, overuse and a host of other factors can cause these fibres to stick together, making movement stiff and sore. Rolling your thumb, fingers, knuckles or elbows across the grain of the muscles starts to separate the fibres, releasing the chemical glue that binds them. Cross-fibre massage can feel as though you are popping across taut ropes, but don't worry: this helps to relax and soften them. Soreness is common during and after cross-fibre work, but be careful not to overdo it. Friction that's applied too quickly or too deeply can injure the tissue. The rule of thumb is: the deeper you go, the slower you go.

energy holds

An energy hold is a simple but powerful massage stroke that you use to send energy to your partner. A still energy hold involves simply resting one or both hands on or near the skin's surface without moving while you breathe and imagine sending energy through your hands (for example, a still hold may be used to initiate or end a massage). A rocking energy hold alternates stillness with rocking, sending waves of energy throughout the body (for example, see the lower back energy hold on page 62 ▶). For centuries, healing practitioners of many cultures have used energy holds to relax a person and to help balance that person's energy while relieving pain and speeding healing.

awaken

Seizing each day and living your life to its fullest takes preparation, both mental and physical. But sometimes it's hard just to get out of bed. Perhaps the best way to begin is by waking up your senses: stir your energy, massage your body and set your mood straight with a grateful heart. You've been given the gift of a new day.

key benefits

▸ Stimulates brain and body

▸ Boosts energy levels

▸ Prepares you for a vibrant day

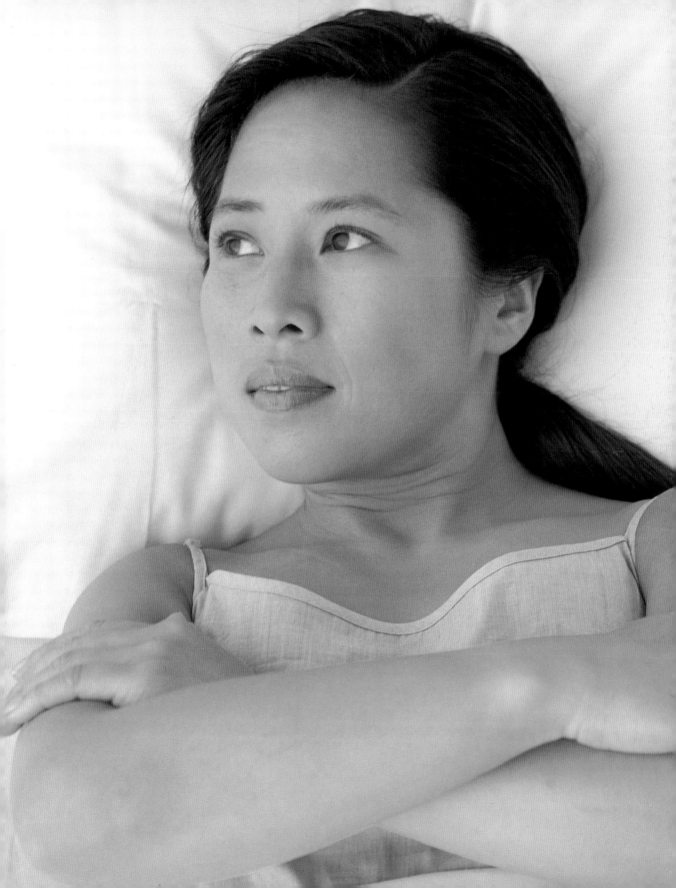

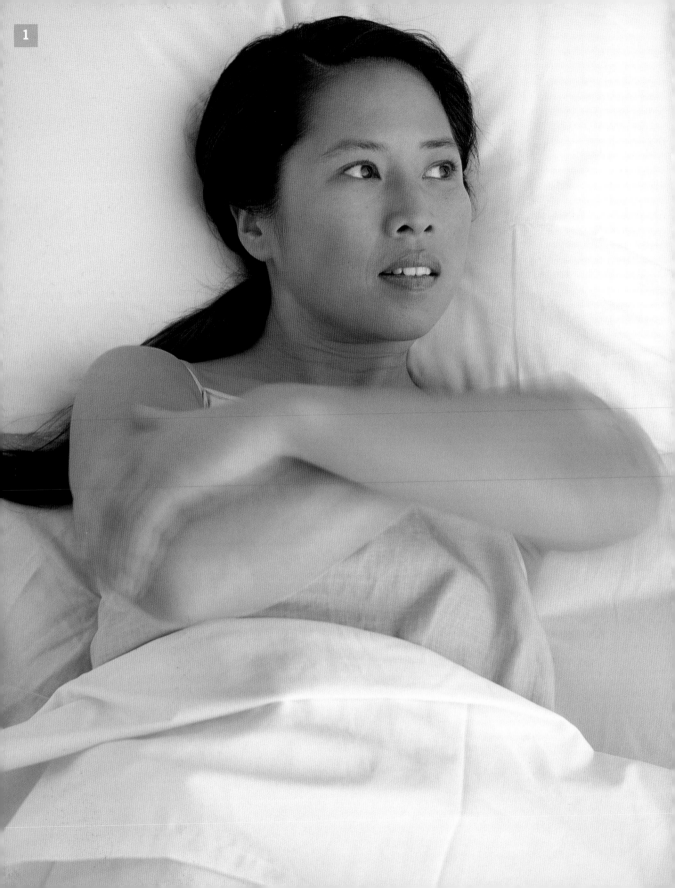

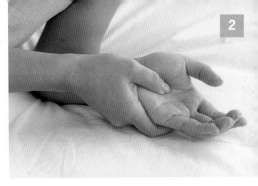

shine and rise

Switch off the alarm and tune into your body. With reflexology and a few quick strokes of self-massage, you can kick-start your day before you stir from bed.

1 arm sweeps

Breathe in deeply and imagine your breath moving energetically through your body from head to toe and back up again. When it reaches your hands on its way back up, cross your arms and briskly rub your hands up and down your arms six times, from wrists to shoulders. According to Chinese medicine, this motion will help stimulate the flow of energy to the heart, lungs and digestive system.

2 palm and finger press

To awaken your resting organs, stimulate the reflexology points that connect with them by pressing deeply into your palm with the thumb of the opposite hand, working friction circles from the wrists to the bases of each finger. Cover the palm's entire surface. To stimulate energy meridians and reflexology points for your head, press, circle and glide along each finger to its tip. Work both hands.

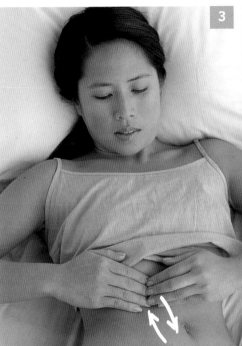

3 belly rub

To jump-start your digestive system, gently sink your fingertips into your lower abdomen about halfway between your navel and the high point of your right hip. Press in and make small, deep clockwise circles, moving up from your right hip to the bottom of your right ribs. Then, staying below the ribs, make clockwise circles across to your left side, then from the left ribs down to the left hip, pushing downwards. At the left hip, make six deep clockwise circles.

4 ear slide

Reflexologists believe that you can awaken energy throughout the body by stimulating points on your ears. With your index finger behind one ear and three fingers in front of it, vigorously slide your hand up and down ten times; then rub the other ear.

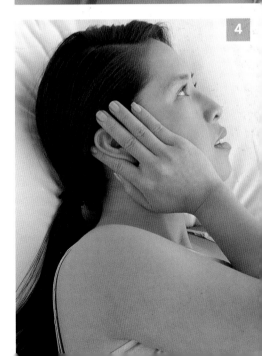

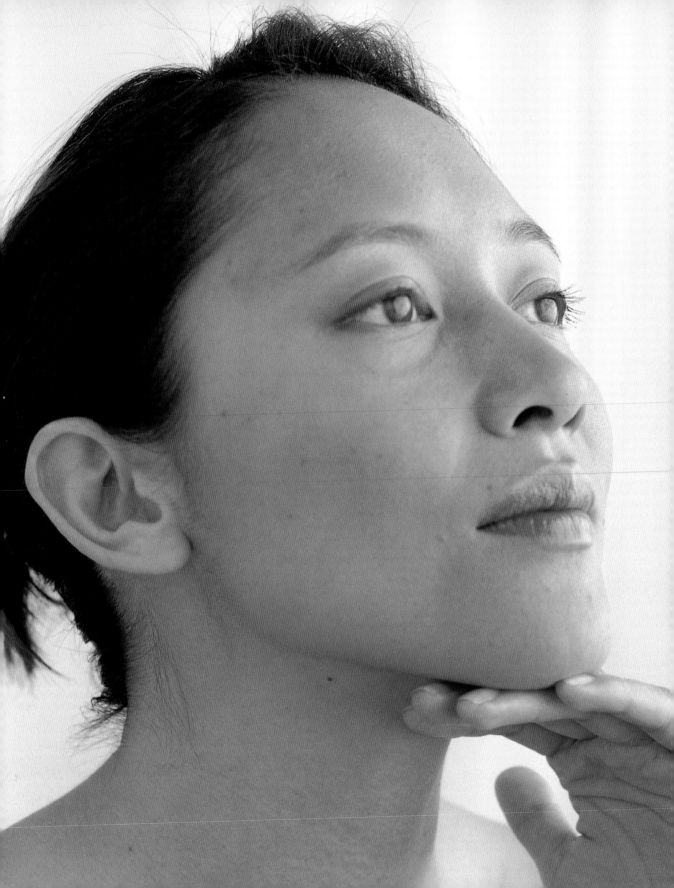

reflect

Your face expresses your heart and reflects your soul, so it deserves special care. Facial expressions affect how the whole body feels, and a quick face massage can brighten both your look and your mood, relieving tension and stress and shifting muscles out of habitual positions. Give your face a lift and let it glow.

key benefits

▶ Helps keep skin taut

▶ Brightens your expression

▶ Elevates your mood

reflect

face forwards

Facial massage helps keep your face toned and revs up energy levels throughout your body. Treat yourself to this routine for head-to-toe benefits.

1 temple circles

Fingertip pressure on your temples can help relieve facial tension. With relaxed hands, gently circle up and back with your middle fingers pressed into the indented areas at the outside edges of your eyebrows. Breathe deeply as you continue circling for three full breaths.

2 cheekbone circles

Starting at the sides of your nostrils, gently press and circle with your middle fingers. Circle, spot by spot, along the contours of the bottom of your cheekbones towards your ears.

3 chin circles

Placing your middle fingers between your lower lip and chin, press firmly and circle with your fingertips, moving outwards and upwards along the jawbone and into the jaw muscles.

4 forehead sweeps

With your middle fingers, gently sweep three times from between your brows to your temples, first above, then below your eyebrows. Then sweep a path from between your brows up to your hairline and across, following your hairline down to your temples. Repeat this sequence three times. Forehead sweeps can also be done while cleansing or moisturising your face. They will tone your muscles and stimulate energy meridians and points that connect to the rest of your body.

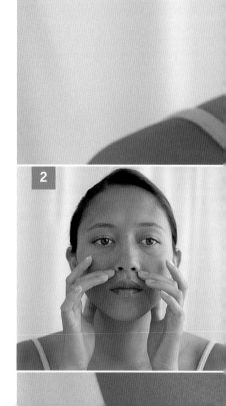
2

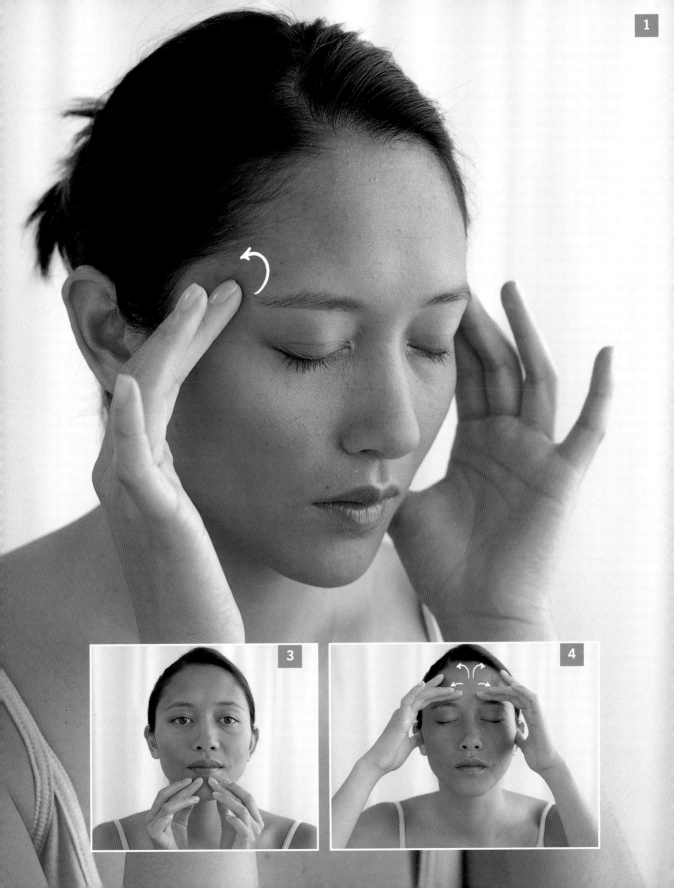

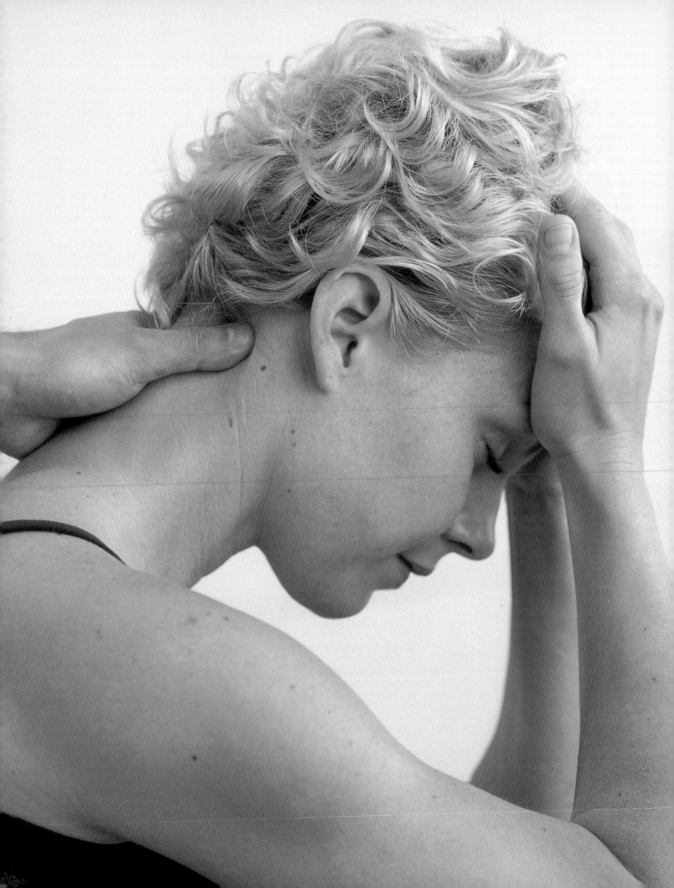

unwind

We all know the feeling: stress and tension give us a pain in the neck. How you view the world, literally and figuratively, affects your neck, so poor posture or off-balance hips – even rigid thinking – can create kinks. Whether you do it yourself or rope in a friend, relief is at hand with a few simple rubs and stretches. Untie those knots and start seeing things straight again.

key benefits

- ▶ Eases tension in your neck
- ▶ Improves blood flow to the brain
- ▶ Relieves tension headaches

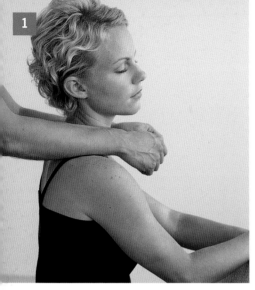

neck nirvana

Enlist an ally to give you a stress-relieving, mind-clearing massage. Sit backwards astride a chair, rest your arms on the back and ask a friend to follow these easy steps.

1 shoulder press

To help ease the tension in your partner's neck, lean your forearms onto her shoulders and press down, increasing the pressure first from one arm, then the other. Then press down with both arms simultaneously as she inhales, lifts her shoulders and holds against the pressure. As she exhales, press back down while she relaxes her shoulders and leans her head from side to side.

2 neck press

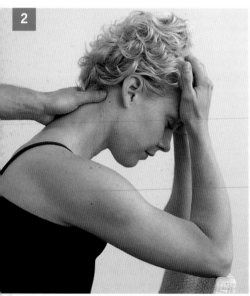

Press deeply with your thumb into the muscles at the base of one side of your partner's skull, sinking your thumb in deeper as she slowly exhales and releasing as she inhales. Work point by point outwards from the muscles beside the spine to about 2.5 cm behind the ear on one side. Repeat on the other side.

3 back-of-neck circles

Holding your partner's forehead with one hand, grip the back of her neck with the other and use circling motions to gently rub across the neck muscles with your thumb and fingers, slowly increasing pressure as the muscles loosen. Do three sets, starting from 2.5 cm below her earlobes and progressing to the base of her neck. Then move in towards the spine and repeat on the muscles on either side of your partner's spine (never press directly on the spine).

4 scalp scrub

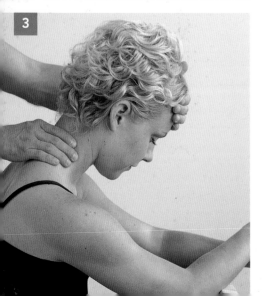

Tightness in the small muscles of the scalp can increase head and neck tension. With both hands, scrub slowly and deeply through your partner's hair, as if you were shampooing it. Start from the base of her skull and work your way over the surface of her scalp until you cover every centimetre.

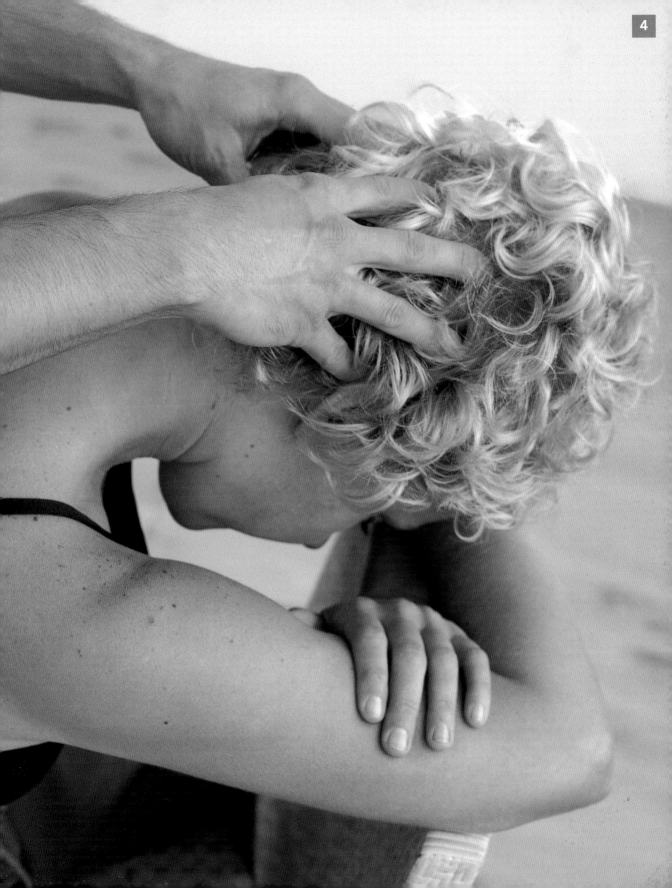

stay loose

If no one is on hand to help you unwind, you can tackle neck stiffness and soreness yourself. Try this sequence of rubs and stretches for quick relief, always being sure to work both sides of your neck.

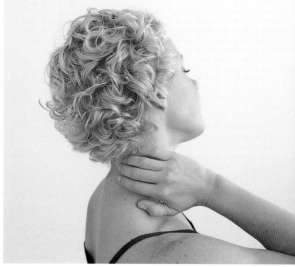

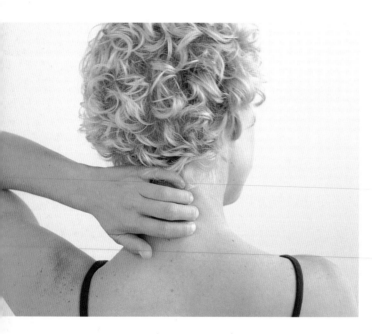

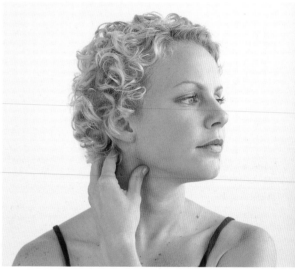

1 extensor circles

Find your extensor muscles (which run parallel to the spine) and make deep finger circles into them from the base of your skull to your shoulders. Then press your fingers in, hold and turn your head from side to side five times, feeling the muscles roll under your fingers.

2 side cross-fibre rub

Press your fingertips into the side of your neck and turn your head back and forth five times. Then rub back and forth across the muscles, from below the earlobe down to the shoulder.

3 neck press

Turn your head to find your sternocleidomastoid muscle. Grasp it firmly about 2.5 cm above your collarbone, and slowly turn your head side to side three times. Repeat, starting 2.5 cm higher.

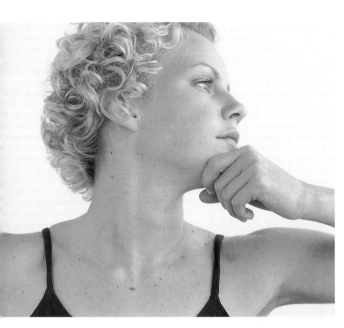

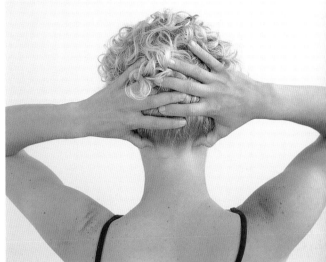

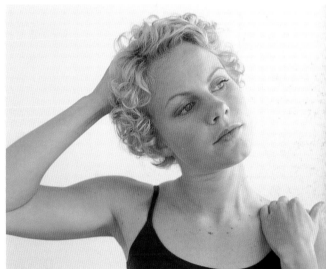

4 neck stretch

While grasping something stable (such as a desk or tabletop) with your right hand, turn your head as far to the left as is comfortable. Then give the front neck muscles a good stretch by using your left hand to gently guide your chin a bit further to the left. Hold this stretch for a few deep breaths.

5 neck circles

Press thumbs in firmly and circle along the base of the skull, beginning on either side of the spine and working out towards the ears. For sore points, hold the pressure as you breathe deeply for three breaths.

6 side stretch

Put your left hand on your left shoulder and use the other hand to guide your head gently towards your right shoulder. Feel the muscles in your neck lengthen as you take three or four deep breaths.

release

Life's tensions tend to collect in our shoulders. If the
weight of the world is on yours, set it down for a
minute and work out the kinks. Unload your worries
and unshoulder your responsibilities (or at least lighten
your bag or backpack). Massage and exercise can help
free your shoulders to keep them moving easily.

key benefits

▶ Eases shoulder strain

▶ Reduces tension down arm and wrist

▶ Improves posture

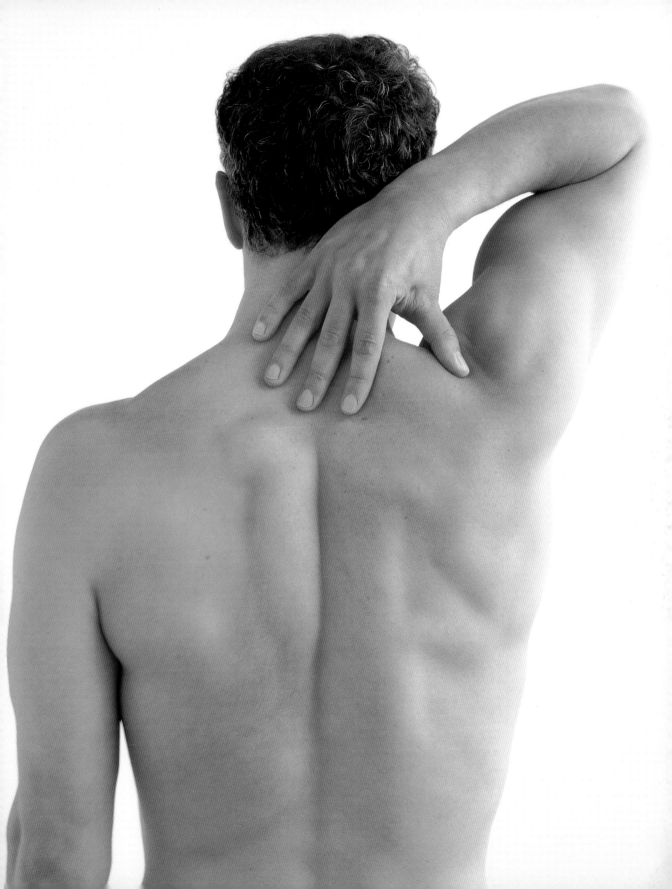

shrug it off

Get into a comfortable position on a chair or floor cushion and ask a friend to join you in these steps designed to straighten out kinks and soothe shoulder aches.

Shield Your Shoulders

- Lighten your load. Every extra gram in your bag, briefcase or backpack can tilt your shoulders and eventually cause muscle pain.
- Keep palms turned inwards as you walk, so shoulders don't round.
- Wear a scarf or turtleneck sweater to protect your neck from cold and draughts, which cause your shoulders to tighten instinctively.
- Soothe your shoulders with scent. Add 5–10 drops of eucalyptus, rosemary, lavender or chamomile essential oil to a bowl of hot water. Soak a towel in the scented water, wring it out and wrap it around your shoulders for 10–20 minutes to help relieve muscle aches.

1 shoulder circles and knead

To relax the muscles between the shoulder blade and spine, lean in with your weight, press into your partner's muscles with your thumbs, glide upwards 2.5 cm and circle back down. Follow the shoulder blade's inner edge, working from the base of the shoulder blade up to the base of the neck. Then use alternating thumbs to knead the muscles along the base of the shoulders and neck.

2 shoulder rub

Cross-fibre massage involves rolling across the grain of muscles to separate their fibres (see page 17 ◄ for more details). Try this technique by bracing one hand on top of your partner's shoulder and using the fingertips of the other hand to rub along the muscles attached to the bottom and outside edge of the shoulder blade, working downwards, parallel to the bone. This area can be tender, so be gentle – but firm enough to not tickle. Repeat on the other side.

3 side sweeps

With your partner's arms raised, massage the shoulder-moving muscles on the side of his ribs, the outer edge of his armpit and along his upper arms. If using massage oil, sweep with long strokes and moderate pressure from his ribs to his elbows and back again. If you're working without oil, press in with your palms and use short back-and-forth rubbing strokes. Work both sides simultaneously.

4 shoulder press

Lean into the tops of your partner's shoulders. With your chin resting on your hands for extra pressure, use your elbows to rub across the fibres into the thick part of his muscles. Lift your elbows and move to another spot. Be sure to stay on muscle – don't press on bone.

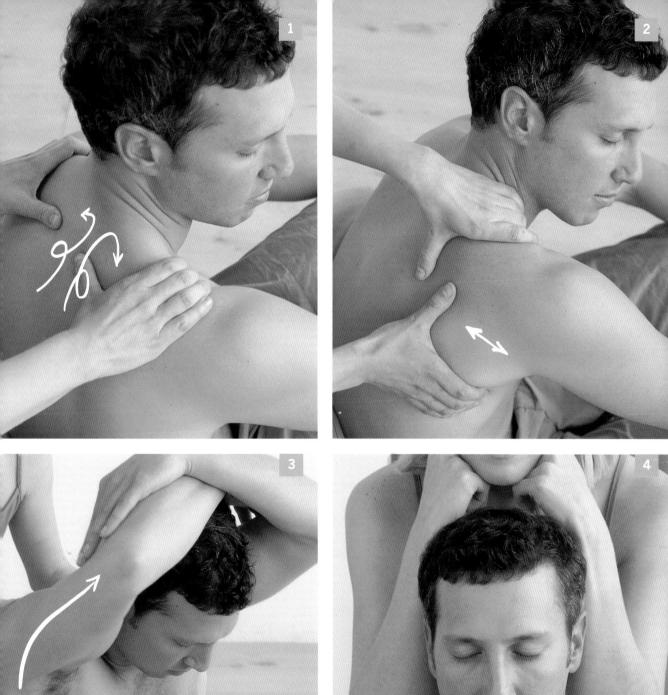
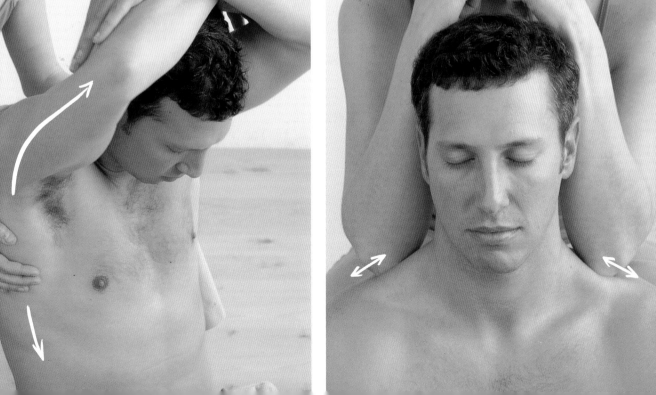

stretch your wings

Exercise and self-massage, done on a regular basis, improve mobility and reduce tension. The trick is to focus on the entire shoulder area, not just the tops, where we feel tension and aches the most.

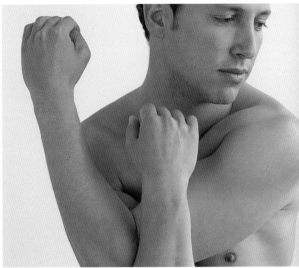

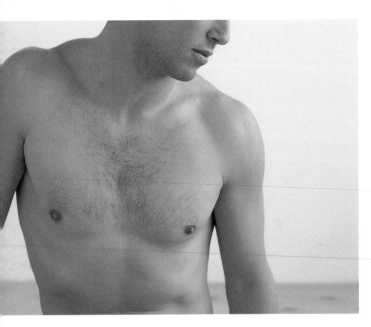

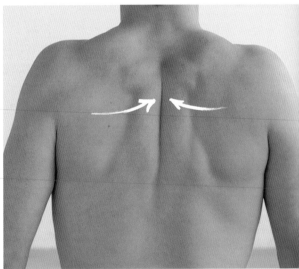

1 shoulder rolls

Lift both shoulders together, aiming for your ears. Hold them up for a full breath, then slowly relax them down; repeat this movement five times. Next roll both shoulders together in circles, first forwards five times, then backwards five times, and finally in alternating circles, five on each side, moving one shoulder at a time.

2 shoulder and arm stretch

With your left arm chest-high and parallel to the ground, slide your right elbow under your left. Pull your left arm towards you and turn your head to the left, stretching the back of your arm and the outside of your shoulder blade. Repeat on your right arm.

3 shoulder blade squeeze

Sometimes the way to loosen muscles is to tighten them first. Pull shoulders back, hold for three breaths, then let them drop and relax. Repeat.

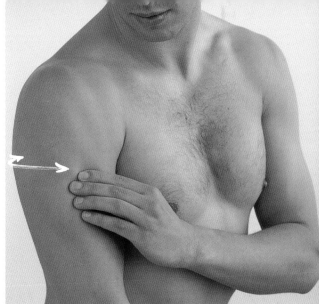

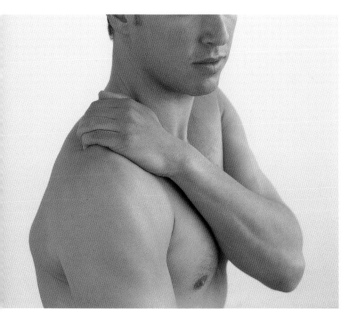

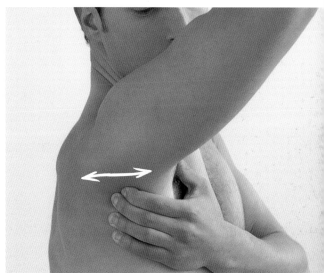

4 shoulder hold

Squeeze as much of your upper shoulder muscles as you can grasp and hold them for 45–90 seconds. Release your grip very, very slowly. This may seem like a long time, but a forced shortening of the muscles tricks the brain into relaxing long-held tension. Work both sides.

5 upper arm cross–fibre rub

Massage the top third of your upper arm: press in firmly and rub back and forth across the muscles, working from the back of your arm to the front.

6 underarm cross–fibre rub

With one arm resting on your head, use the other to reach across your chest and feel for the bottom corner of your shoulder blade. Sink your fingertips in and rub back and forth across the muscles along the edge of the bone, working up to your shoulder.

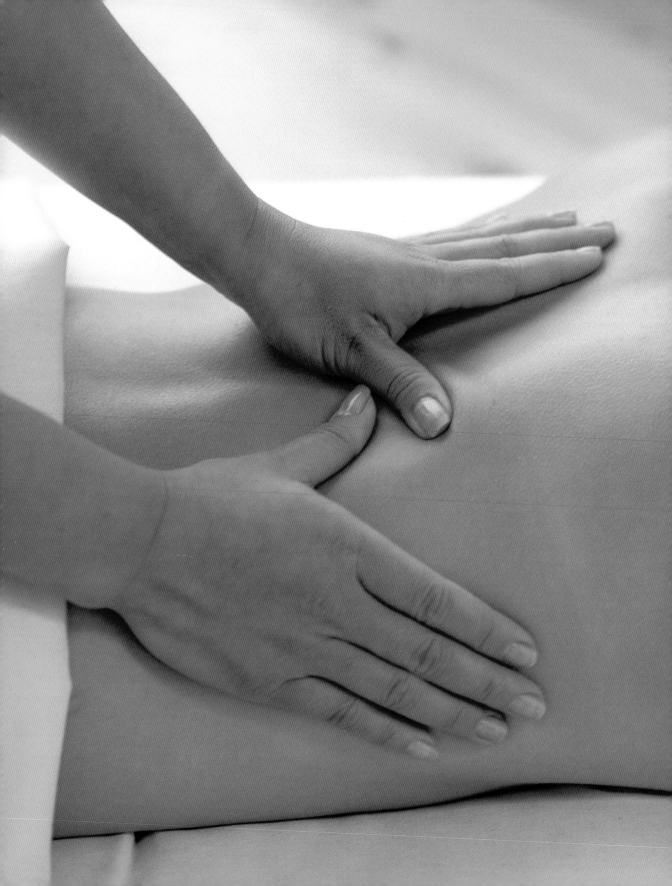

relax

Back pain is all too familiar to most of us. Stress gathers in tight muscles, and long hours of sitting only make it worse. That's why good back care is one of the best gifts you can give a friend – or yourself. Deep massage and energy holds with a partner are amazingly potent; there are also effective ways to help yourself when you are on your own.

key benefits

► Loosens up back muscles

► Reduces stress

► Helps alleviate back pain

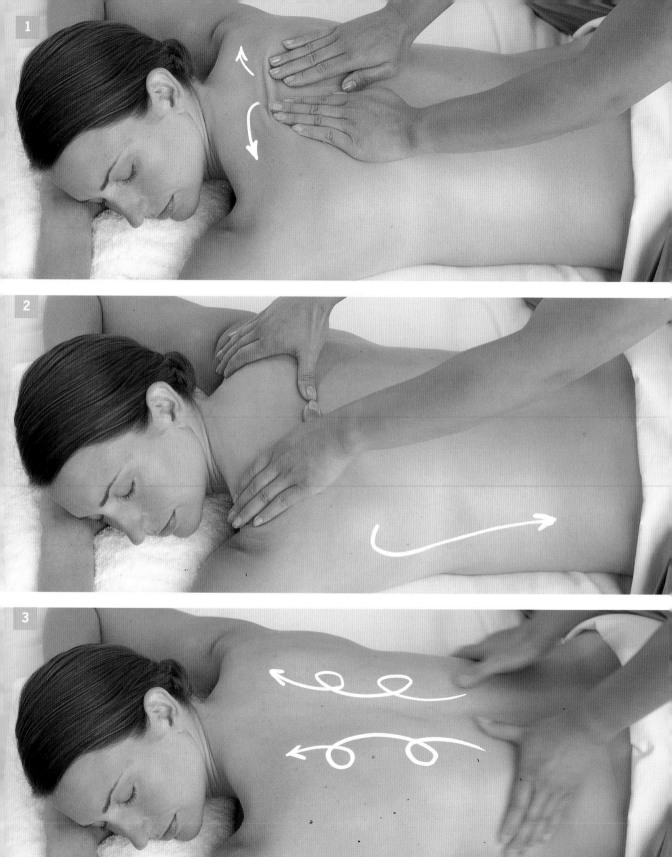

back to basics

Lie on a firm, comfortable surface covered with a sheet to add cosiness and to soak up stray massage oil. Relax and ask a friend to work your back with these easy steps.

1 spine glide

Warm some massage oil in your hands, then glide up the thick muscles along the sides of your partner's spine, first just to spread the oil, then using subsequent strokes to work more deeply. Pressing in with your fingertips, glide up the curve of her lower back, contouring your hands to her back muscles as you continue up to the base of her neck. Keep your fingertips together as you glide.

2 shoulder fan and sweep and stretch

Finish a spine glide and, at the base of her neck, fan your hands out and stroke across the top and down the sides of your partner's shoulders. Curve around and pull down towards her ribs. Continue gliding down her sides towards her hips, sweep your fingers under her waist, lean back and gently pull, stretching her lower back. Reposition your hands on her lower back and repeat the sequence – spine glide, shoulder fan and sweep and stretch – four more times. Reapply oil as necessary, but don't make the skin too slippery.

3 thumb circles and rocking energy hold

Starting at the lower back, press your thumbs into the muscles on either side of her spine. Using heavy pressure, circle your thumbs into the muscles as you work up to the neck. Knead your fingers into the muscles around the base of her neck and across her shoulders.

To finish this back massage, sit beside your partner and place one hand on her tailbone and your other hand at the base of her neck. Rock her hips from side to side with your lower hand for 20 seconds, then be still for 20 seconds. Repeat the cycle for several minutes until your partner's breathing becomes deep and regular.

Back-Care Tips
- For muscle pain, lie on the floor with a tennis ball under a sore spot, and roll gently across the ball. Or put two tennis balls in a sock and position it so that a ball is on either side of your spine; roll up and down.
- Deep breathing (expanding the ribs fully) helps prevent back pain.
- At work, knead sore spots by placing your fist between your back and a chair. Lean into your knuckles and rock from side to side.
- Apply a cold pack (a bag of frozen peas also works well) to painful spots for 10–15 minutes.

kick back

These moves massage and exercise leg, hip and abdominal muscles that indirectly cause back problems. Perform them on a soft surface. And for sharp or chronic back pain, seek professional help.

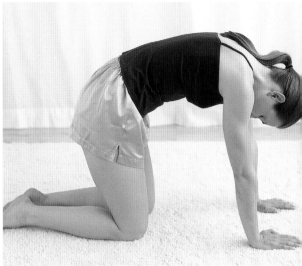

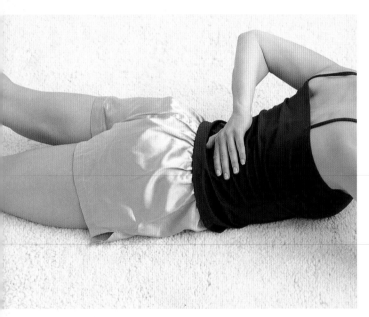

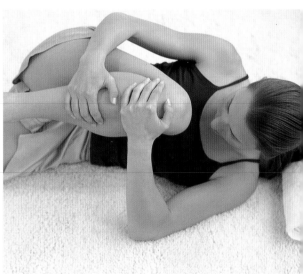

1 back release

To relax the thick muscles along your spine (the extensors), lie face down, gently lift your left leg, arch your upper body back and put your hand on your back to feel the muscles contract on the right side of the spine. Hold for ten seconds before slowly lowering both upper body and leg to the floor. Relax. Repeat five times, then switch legs to work the other side of your back.

2 classic cat stretch

Start on your hands and knees, spine parallel to the floor. Breathe in deeply. Exhale as you round your back up and lower your head. Inhale as you arch your back and look up. Repeat four more times.

3 side stretch

Lie on your side and hug the top knee to your chest. Inhale, then exhale and straighten the leg. At the same time, reach your top arm over your head, stretching your waist. Do five times on each side.

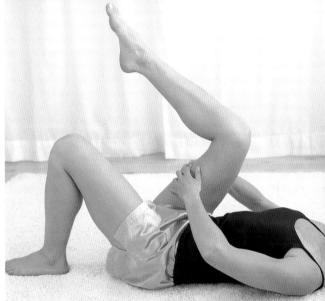

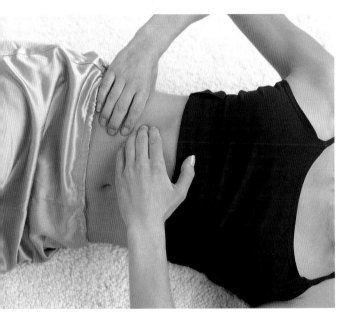

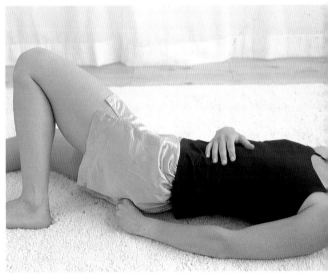

4 side knead

Lie on your side and massage the oblique muscles, which are located at the side of your waist, between your ribs and hips. With your thumbs and fingers, feel for the deep, ropy muscles and knead them gently. For sore or tight spots, pinch firmly and hold any tender point for three full breaths. Repeat on the other side.

5 hamstrings stretch and rub

Inhale deeply. Exhaling, pull your knee towards your chest with your leg as straight as possible; hold for five seconds. Relax, bend your knee and use your fingertips to rub across the hamstring fibres, moving side to side, knee to buttocks. Repeat on other leg.

6 gluteal press

Bend your left knee, raise your left buttock to slip a fist under, then roll around on it. Hold for three breaths on sore spots; then switch legs and repeat.

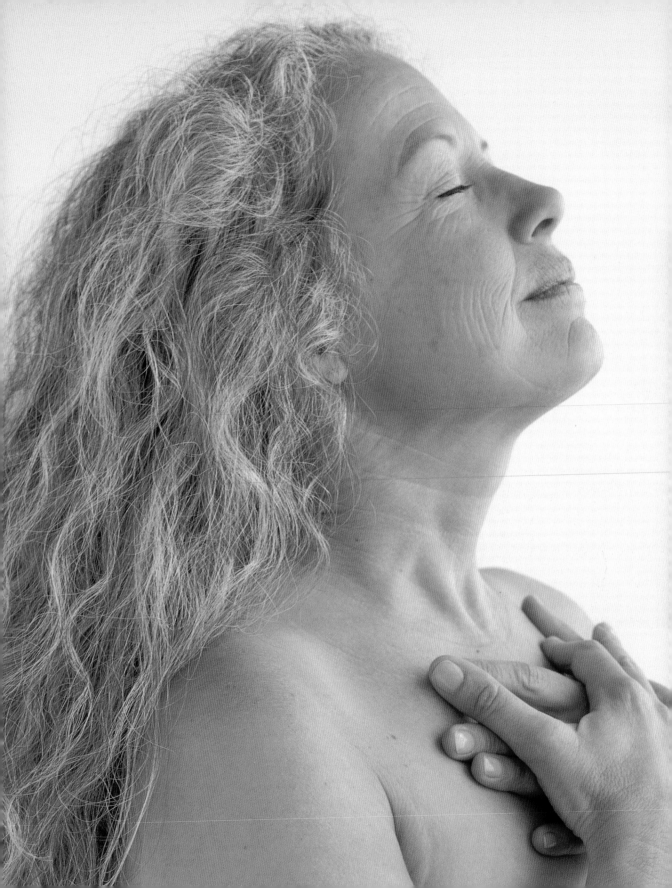

inspire

The way we breathe can be a metaphor for how we live our lives: full, deep and expansive, or tight and shallow. The secret to achieving a life of ample inspiration lies in freeing constriction in our chest, our ribs – and even our thoughts. Out with the bad, in with the good. Take a breather and open yourself up to a broader view of life and its boundless possibilities.

key benefits

- ▶ Releases chest constriction
- ▶ Encourages deep breathing to increase energy
- ▶ Restores enthusiasm and improves your outlook

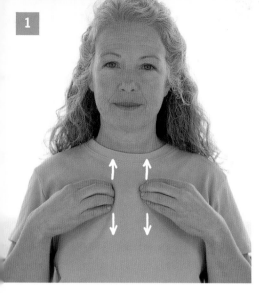

breathe easy

This sequence can be done just about anywhere. Make yourself comfortable, relax for a few moments and savour the feeling of your energy expanding with your breath.

1 breastbone rib rub

Tension can set in where the ribs attach to the breastbone, inhibiting full inhalation. Starting below the collarbones where the ribs join to each side of the breastbone, sink the fingertips of both hands into the space between ribs, then rub up and down over your ribs five times. Move your fingers down a few centimetres and continue rolling across the ribs, working down both sides of the breastbone.

2 side stretches

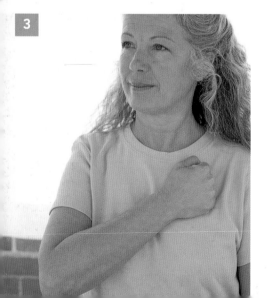

With your right arm overhead, lean to your left, stretching your side muscles. Breathing deeply, rub your right side briskly with light strokes that run from your waist to your armpit. Where you find sore spots, take a moment to rub across the muscle grain using cross-fibre friction (see page 17 ◄ for more about this technique), sinking in your fingertips and rubbing front to back. Repeat on the other side.

3 chest percussion

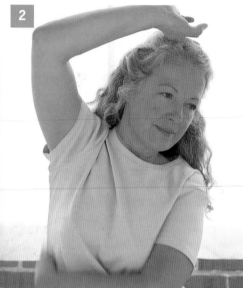

Tapping the chest sharply with loose fists can help loosen congestion in the lungs and stimulate circulation in the chest muscles. Making sure you work only below the collarbone, use your right hand to pound the left side of your chest from breastbone to shoulder. Then use your left hand to do the same on the right side of your chest.

4 chest rub

Find your intercostal muscles, located in the grooves between your ribs. Press in with your index and middle fingers and rub them with short, deep, side-to-side motions. Repeat between as many ribs as you can feel. Then raise one arm over your head (see inset photo) and knead any tight or ropy chest muscles, pressing and rolling them between your thumb and fingers. Repeat on the other side.

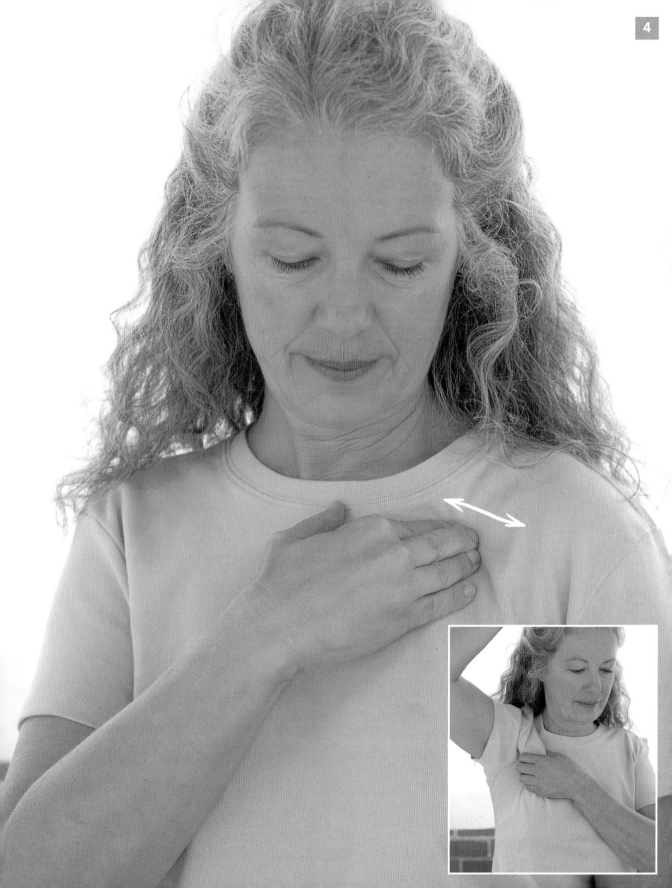

rest

Whether it's too many dishes, mouse clicks or workouts, chances are your hands need a break. Repetitive movements are tiring and can cause long-term damage. Stop for a moment and ease the tension that's built up in your digits. Your hands work hard for you – so treat them with care.

key benefits

▸ Reduces tension in hands, arms and wrists

▸ Releases built-up toxins

▸ Helps stave off repetitive-strain injury

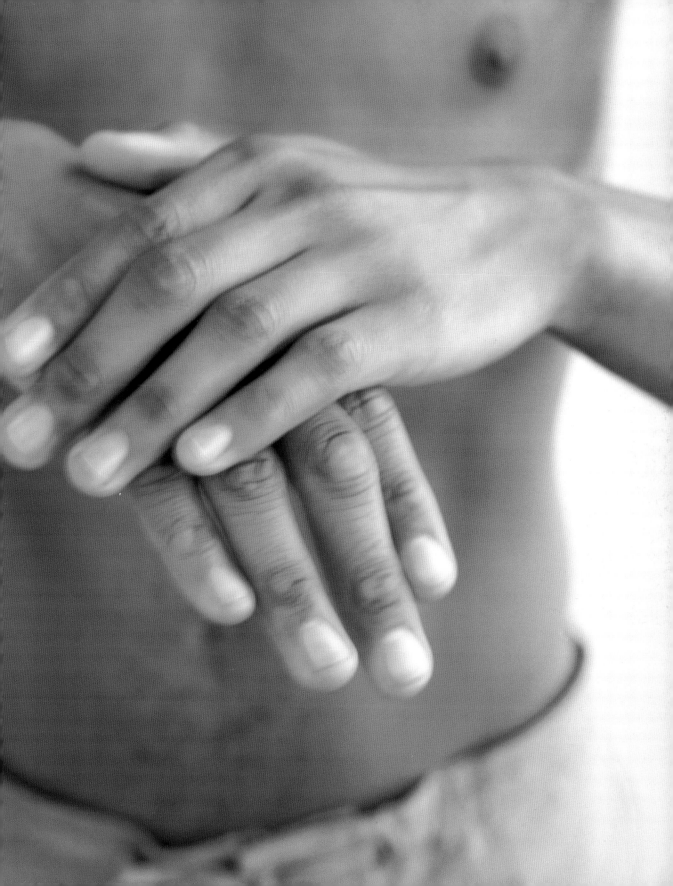

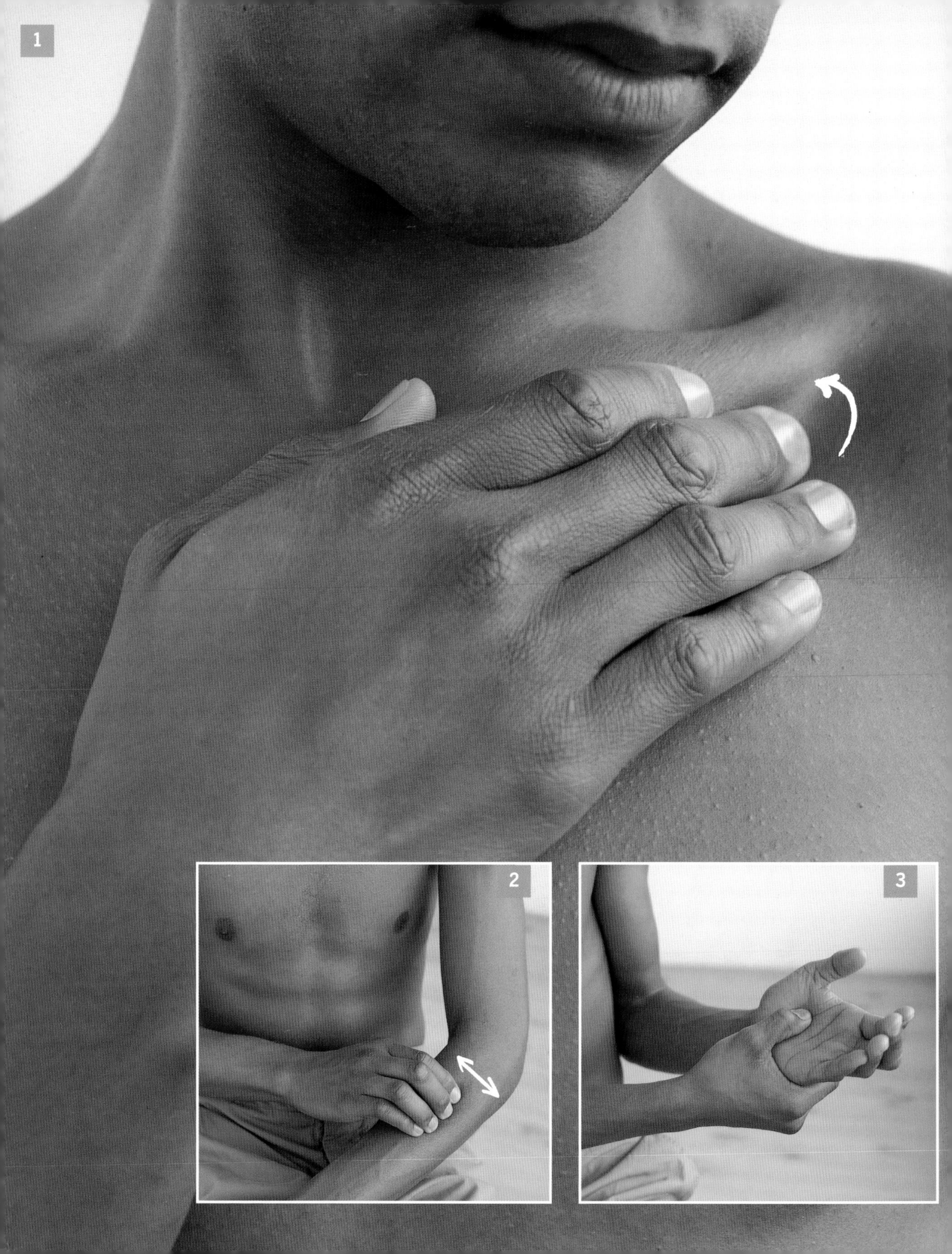
1
2
3

get a grip

Hand, arm and wrist problems are on the increase.
Take care of your hands with these steps designed to
release tension, flush toxins and help banish stress.

1 fluid circles and sweeps

To alleviate arm swelling that can cause pressure on your wrist, circle
lightly with your fingertips along the base of your collarbone, from
shoulder to breastbone. Then sweep your fingers using featherlight
strokes, again inwards along the base of your collarbone. Repeat the
circle and sweep strokes 10–15 times on each side of your chest.

2 cross-fibre rub and release

With firm fingertip pressure, rub horizontally across the muscles on
all the surfaces of your forearm, starting 5 cm above your elbow and
inching downwards to the middle of your forearm (pictured). For
further release, massage the muscles between the two bones in your
forearm in an up-and-down direction. Starting near the wrist, use
your thumb to pull the skin back 5 mm. Press down into the muscle
and slide forwards with medium pressure, lifting and repeating,
working gradually along to the elbow. Repeat on the other arm.

3 hand friction circles

The small muscles in your hands and fingers become tired quickly.
Release tension and built-up toxins within these tiny muscles by
making deep circular-friction strokes with the thumb of your other
hand. Cover your palm and the length of each finger, starting with
the thumb and ending with the little finger. When you come across a
sore point, pause, press in for 10–15 seconds, then release and move on.

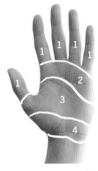

Reflexology Hand Basics
Reflexologists believe that
pressing into key points in
specific zones in your hands
helps activate and balance the
energy that keeps organs and
specific areas of the body
healthy. The body has lines of
energy that end in specific zones
in your hand: zone 1 in the
fingers connects to the head and
neck; zone 2 links with the chest
and lungs; zone 3 corresponds to
the organs above the navel; zone
4 links to the digestive tract and
the area below the navel. (See
page 59 ▸ for information about
foot reflexology zones.)

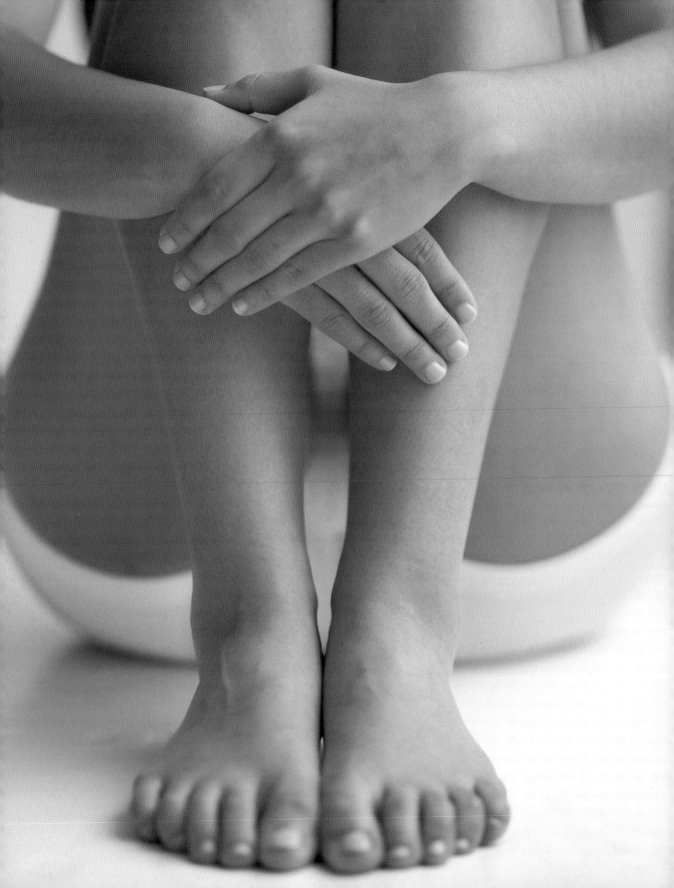

loosen

Legs can get overworked from too much exercise or weak from a sedentary lifestyle. Flexible legs are your number-one vehicle for life's journey, and massage can help improve circulation, lengthen muscles and work out sore spots before they become chronic. You've still got a long way to go, so stay active – by keeping loose.

key benefits

▶ Lengthens tight muscles

▶ Stimulates circulation

▶ Eases soreness

get a leg up

Whether from too much or too little exercise, legs can feel weary, sore and in need of attention. Put your leg up on a friend's lap and ask her to follow these steps.

1 calf knead

Sitting on a couch, a chair or the floor, rest your partner's leg in your lap and support his knee so it bends a little. Knead into the calf muscles with alternating hands, using rounded fingers held closely together, gripping and rolling the muscles from knee to mid-shin. To make your hands glide more easily, use massage oil.

2 shin circles

Sink your thumbs gently but firmly into the thick muscles on the outside edge of your partner's shin-bone and circle deeply, working down along the bone from knee to ankle.

3 knee circles

Place your thumbs together on the inside edge of your partner's kneecap and press in firmly but gently. Circle your thumbs around the kneecap in opposite directions until they meet on the outer side.

4 thigh pulls

With your palms contoured to the muscles on the inside of your partner's thigh, pull each hand towards you with overlapping sweeps, using medium pressure and keeping your fingers together. Begin the strokes just above the knee and work rhythmically up the thigh.

5 thigh knead

Grasp the top of your partner's thigh between your thumbs and fingers and knead it firmly, squeezing and rolling the muscles as if wringing a towel. Work from above the knee to the top of the thigh. Repeat on the inner thigh. Then do this sequence on the other leg.

Liberate Your Legs

- Being a "lady" can be bad for your legs. High heels hurt your feet, knees and back; wearing hosiery or crossing your legs at the knee cuts off circulation; and tight skirts limit walking strides. Change your wardrobe and liberate your legs!
- To stimulate leg circulation, mix 5–10 drops of eucalyptus, orange or rosemary essential oil with 5 teaspoons of massage oil and stroke vigorously into leg muscles.
- Let gravity help tired legs. To reduce swelling and help speed up circulation, lie on your back on the floor and put your legs straight up against a wall for a few minutes.

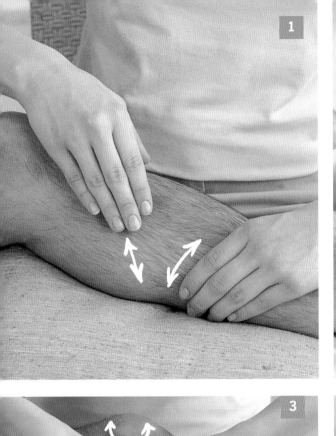

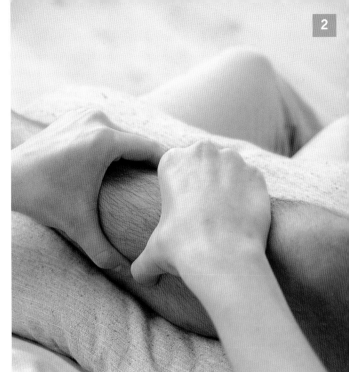

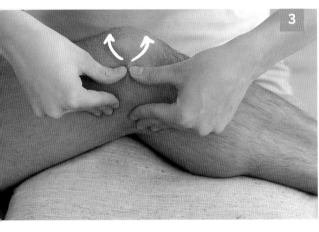

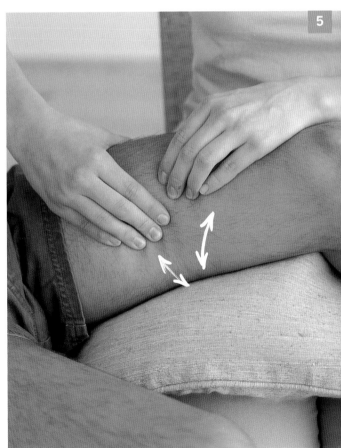

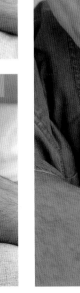

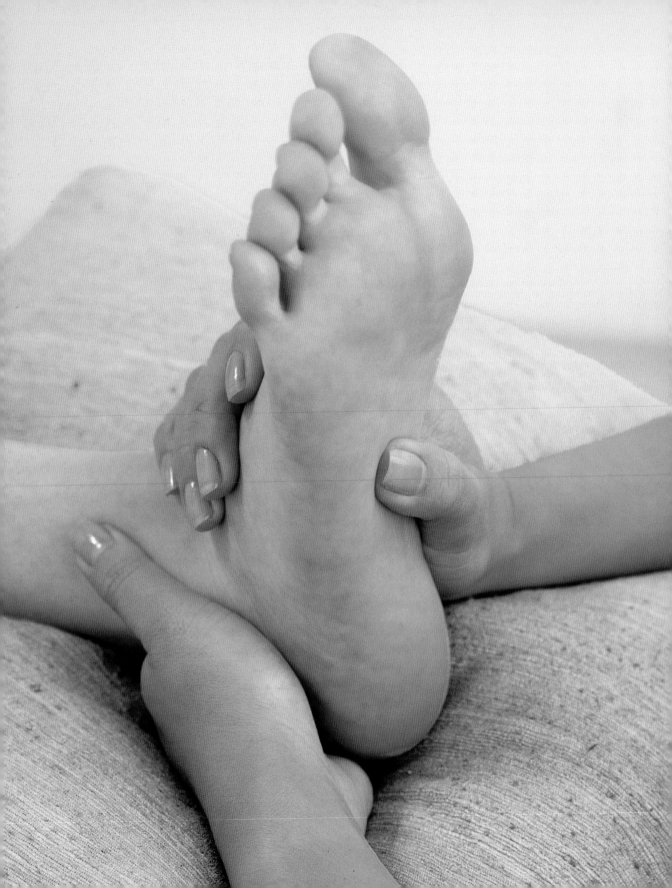

soothe

Our poor feet: shoved into shoes, hoisted into heels, trotted to and fro, standing for everything but our principles – no wonder they kick up a fuss. Free them from their fashion prisons, soak them in the bath and treat them to a rub. A foot massage is one of life's great pleasures and works miracles, not only on tired feet but also on our general wellbeing.

key benefits

► Comforts aching feet

► Works reflexology energy zones

► Revives sagging spirits

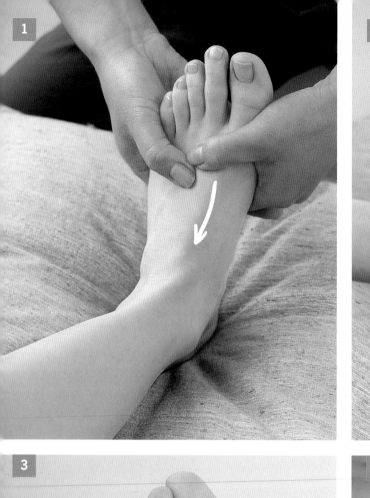

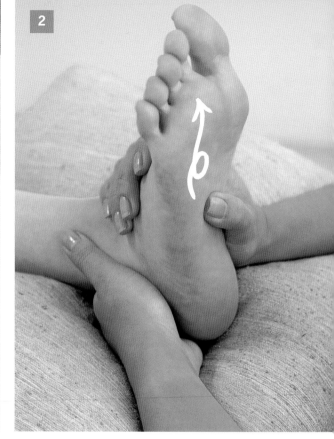

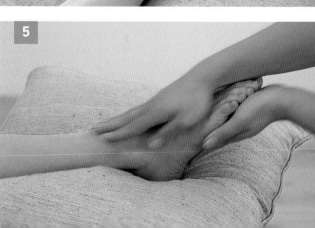

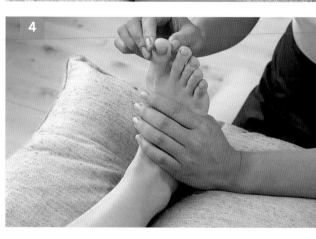

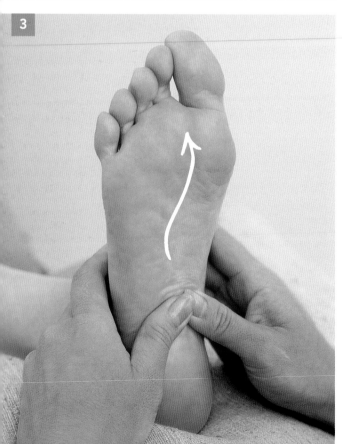

sole salvation

Get a friend to help you cool your heels. Rest your
foot on a firm cushion opposite her and ask her
to follow these steps on one foot, then the other.

1 groove glides
Put your dominant hand, palm up, in your other hand and place
the edges of your index fingers against the sole of your partner's
foot. Place your thumbs at the juncture of the big and second toes,
pressing with thumbs and fingers, and slide down the groove
between the bones from toes to ankle. Lightly slide back up, move
across to another juncture and repeat three more times.

2 arch circles
Make deep, overlapping thumb circles over the entire surface of your
partner's heel and arch. Then place your thumb just above the arch
and press into the groove between the bones that lead up to the
second and big toes. Working outwards, circle with your thumb up
each groove, circling from the top of the instep towards each toe.

3 sole glides
With your thumbs braced side by side for firm pressure, glide up the
sole of the foot from the middle of the heel, up through the grooves
in the ball of the foot, to between the toes. Ease the pressure and
slide back to the heel. Repeat two more times.

4 toe wiggles
Massage each toe, pressing your thumb and index finger together
and circling from base to tip. Next, wiggle each toe backwards,
forwards and around in circles, starting with small circles and spiralling
into bigger ones (take care to ensure you're not causing any pain).

5 foot sweep
For a soothing finish, contour and press your hands together on the
top and bottom of her foot. Pull both your hands off the toes and
towards you, then repeat these steps two more times.

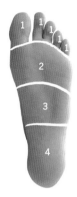

Reflexology Foot Basics
Reflexologists believe that the feet
have zones that, when pressed,
affect corresponding zones in the
body. For example, the toes (zone 1)
link with the head and neck, and
the ball of the foot (zone 2) links
to the chest and shoulders. The area
from below the ball of the foot to the
middle of the arch (zone 3) connects
to the organs beneath the ribs but
above the navel, while the area
from the middle of the foot to
the heel (zone 4) corresponds
to the lower abdomen and pelvis.
(See page 51 ◄ for information
about hand reflexology zones.)

connect

When life gets too hectic, we sometimes find ourselves

neglecting even our most cherished relationships.

A full-body massage offers a splendid opportunity to

reconnect with each other, bringing pleasure to both

giver and receiver. So caress forgotten curves, stroke

away soreness – and discover one another anew.

key benefits

- ▶ Soothes stressed muscles
- ▶ Lets you give and receive pleasure
- ▶ Helps you get closer to your partner

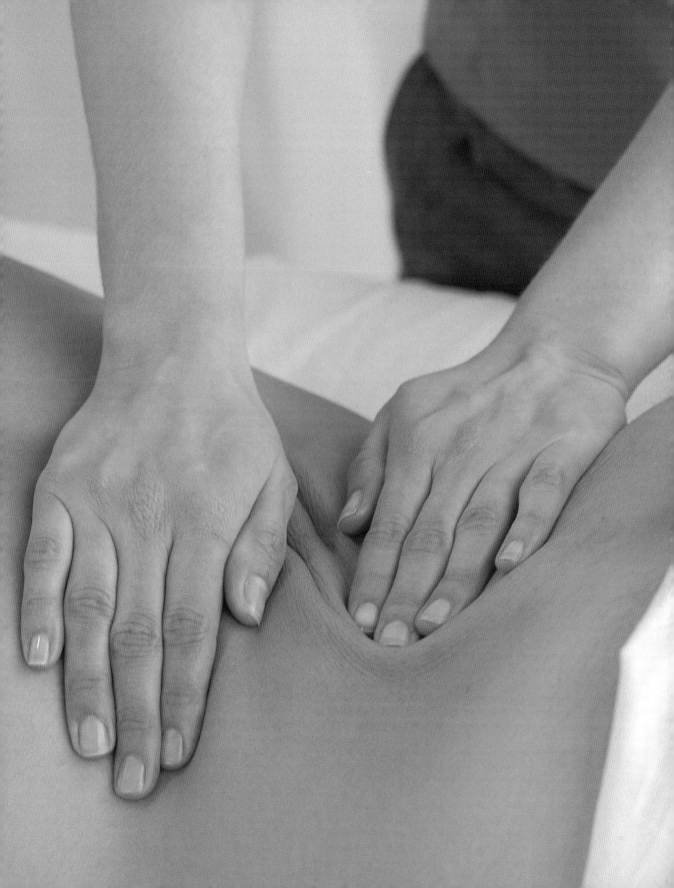

take care

Get your partner to lie on a surface that provides strong support, adding a pillow under his head if it's more comfortable. Then follow these steps to bodily bliss.

1 back glide

Warm massage oil in your hands and spread it thinly over your partner's back and sides. Then press your hands along either side of his spine and glide them from his shoulders to his lower back, keeping your fingertips together and using moderate pressure. At his waist, fan out your hands, swinging your fingers down along his sides, and pull back up along his waist and ribs. Repeat several times.

2 back knead

Rest your hands on your partner's lower back, then bend your left knee and push your left hand across his back while pulling your right hand towards you. (Protect your own back by rocking your weight as you reach.) When your strokes reach opposite sides of his waist, press in firmly and drag your hands back to the centre. Then bend your right knee, push your right hand across, and pull your left hand back. Repeat this criss-cross motion on the back ten times.

3 shoulder and buttock knead

Reach across your partner's back and knead the muscles between his spine and shoulder blade, massaging along the edge of his shoulder blade. Then reach across his back, sink your fingertips into the far side of the gluteal muscles of his buttocks, lean back and pull towards his tailbone with alternating hands. Do this ten times on one side, then walk around him and repeat these steps on his other side.

4 lower back energy hold

Hold your hands together above your partner's lower back for a moment. Then lightly set them on his back and rock back and forth very gently. Alternate between rocking and stillness. Feel for any sense of warmth or tingling – signs of pent-up energy being released. After 3–5 full breaths, slowly lift your hands off his back.

Aromatherapy Massage Oils

- To create your own aromatherapy massage oil blend, mix 10 drops of essential oil with 50 ml of a carrier oil such as sweet almond, grapeseed, sesame or jojoba oil.
- To soothe and relax, try lavender or chamomile essential oil.
- For a vigorous massage, opt for stimulating essential oils such as rosemary or peppermint.
- For more aromatherapy massage oil recipes, see page 13 ◄.

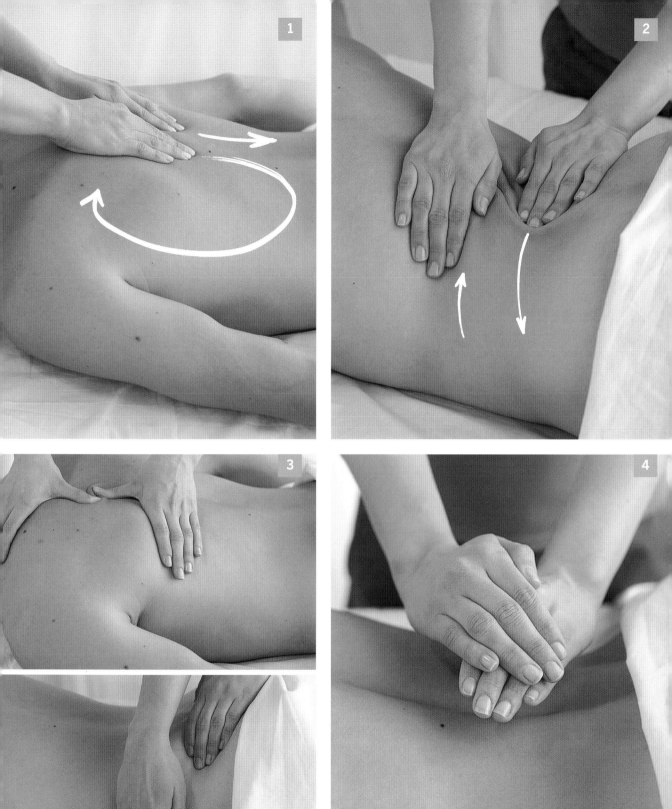

talk touch

Follow the Platinum Rule of Massage: do unto others as they want done unto them. Take time to discuss touch preferences. And be sure to work both your partner's arms and legs in this soothing sequence.

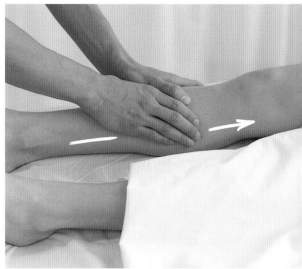

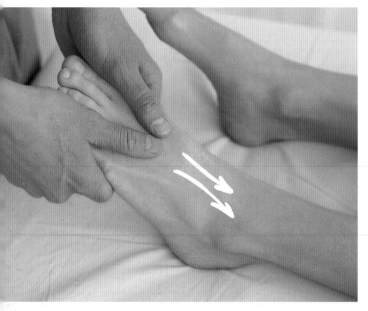

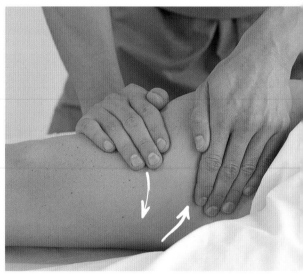

1 foot strokes

Massage both surfaces of the feet, trying different hand positions, strokes and pressures. Start off with a downward gliding stroke, pressing your thumbs into the top of your partner's foot and your fingers into the sole.

2 leg glides

Starting at the ankle, press in with your fingers and thumbs and glide up to the knee. Then glide from knee to hip, sweeping along the thigh muscles halfway up, then out towards the hipbone.

3 thigh wringing

Wring the thigh muscles by simultaneously pushing and pulling with alternating hands. Alternately bend your knees to protect your back as each palm moves low on her inner thigh. Work each thigh six times.

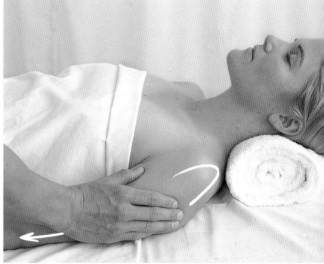

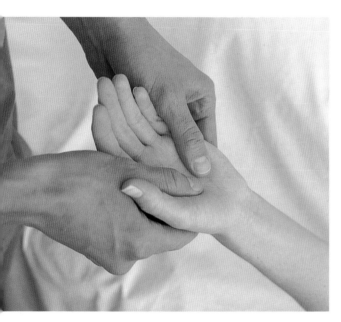

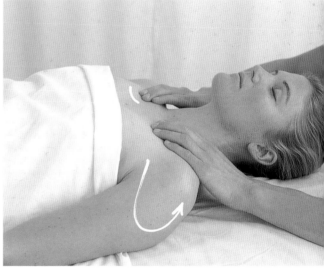

4 hand circles

Open your partner's palm and use both hands to massage into it with thumb circles, covering the entire surface. Circle up her thumb and fingers from base to tip, pressing and rubbing them firmly between your thumbs and index fingers.

5 arm glides

Stabilise your partner's forearm with your left hand and, with your right, wrap your fingers and thumb around her forearm; then press in and glide up to her shoulder. Curve around the shoulder and glide lightly back down her arm, repeating five times.

6 chest sweeps

With fingers flat on the breastbone, sweep across the chest to the shoulders, then sweep under them and up to the base of the skull. Repeat five times.

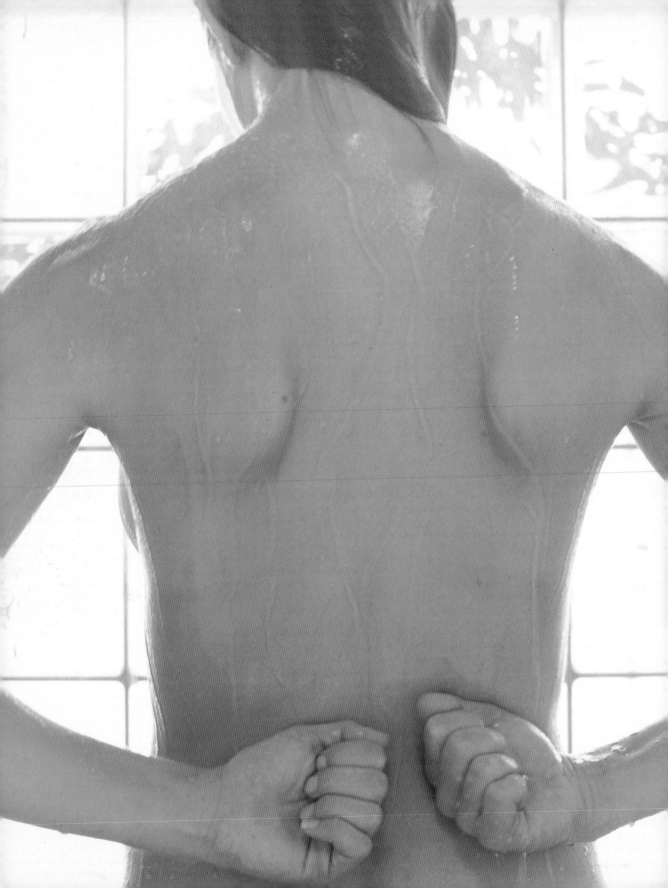

repair

If you've been a bit immoderate, rescue yourself with some hangover helpers that also help kick-start your energy meridians. Mother Nature may take her time clearing up foggy heads and rumbly stomachs, but a hot shower and some detoxing massage can speed up the process considerably. Let the healing begin.

key benefits

▶ Relieves headaches and nausea

▶ Speeds up detoxification

▶ Wakes up a sluggish system

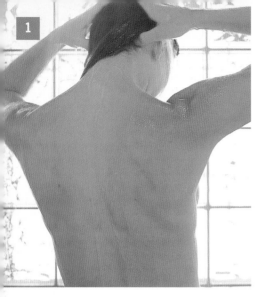

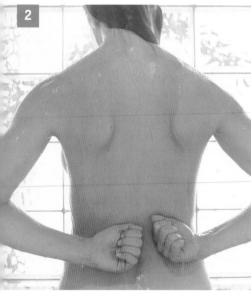

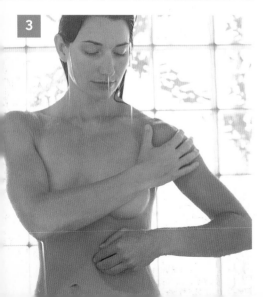

get clear

Feeling groggy the morning after? Hop into a steaming shower and revive your sluggish system with these simple routines designed to get you back on track.

1 skull press

To help relieve nausea and headaches, press your thumbs into the muscles and acupressure points along the base of your skull and neck. Starting where the back of your head meets your neck, place your thumbs on each side of the spine, press in for two breaths, release, move a couple of centimetres sideways and repeat, moving outwards to 2.5 cm behind the ears. Return to the spine, press in on each side again and work your thumbs downwards along your neck.

2 kidney percussion

Give your detoxification filters a hand by gently pummelling your kidneys – located at the base of your ribs – to help break up toxic crystal deposits. Lean over slightly, reach behind you and gently pound below your lower ribs with soft fists. Do each side 12 times.

3 point press

With your fingertips, find a classic acupressure point for relieving hangover symptoms at the bottom edge of your ribcage, directly in line with your nipple. Feel for a slight indentation in the bone there. Once you've found it, press gently upwards into the ribs. Hold the point for ten full breaths. Repeat on the other side.

4 crown release

To help release congested energy in your head, press your palms down on the top of your head and hold for three deep breaths; then circle ten times with your fingertips. Tight, dehydrated scalp muscles can exacerbate headaches; release tension by pulling your hair with three-second tugs all over your scalp.

5 scalp scrub

Scrub over your whole scalp, as if shampooing, with firm pressure. For extra uplift, finish off by washing your hair with a shampoo that has an invigorating scent, such as grapefruit or rosemary.

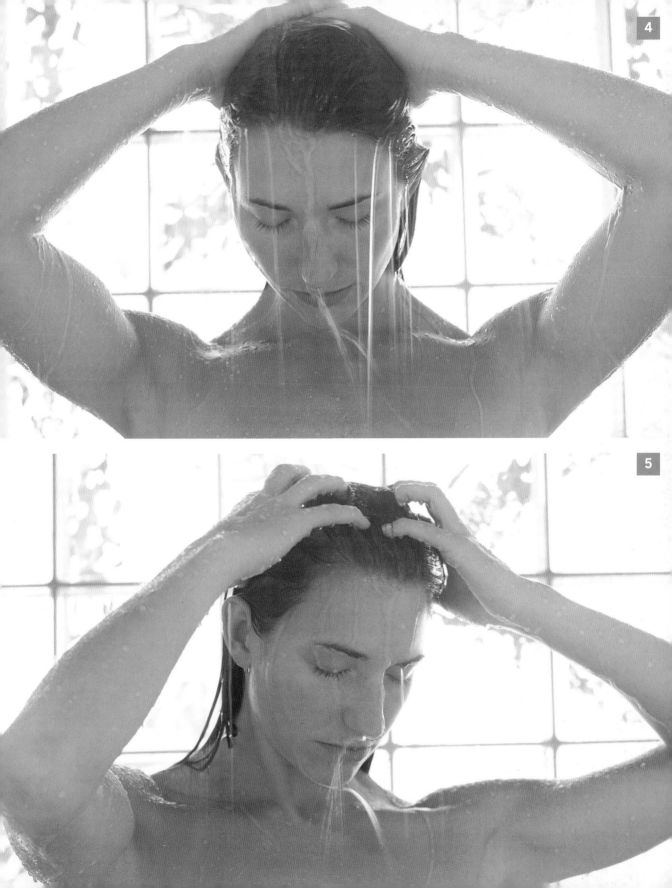

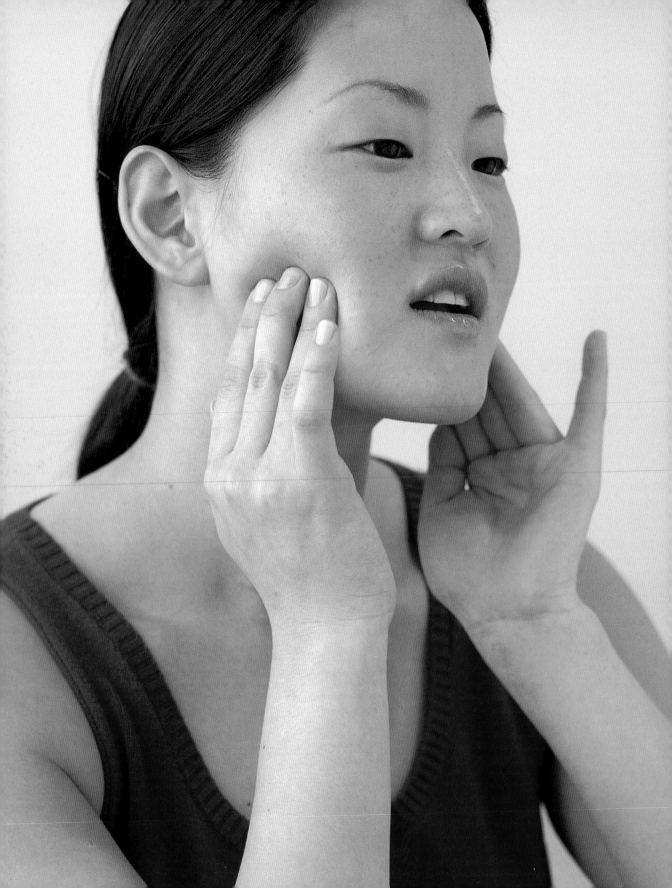

revive

Whether we're raising children, clocking up hours at the office or both, long days sap our energy. We're just not meant to work this hard, so we sometimes run out of steam. If you're drooping and there's no time for a nap, recharge with an energising massage. Stir your spirits, boost your energy – and get back to work.

key benefits

▶ Perks up energy levels

▶ Restores mental focus

▶ Brightens your mood

work wonders

If you feel yourself fading, try these Eastern exercises designed to revitalise energy. The easy moves can shore up sagging spirits and jump-start a bleary brain.

1 arm knocks

In Chinese medicine, energy meridians that affect internal organs run in lines through the arms to the fingers. Stimulate these lines and get an instant boost by knocking them with a loose fist. Gently tap the inside of your arm from armpit to wrist, and then up from the outside of your arm from wrist to shoulder. Then do the other arm.

2 head knocks

To clear your head and focus your thinking, knock lightly all over your head with soft, half-open fists. The lines of the major energy meridians associated with major organs of the body run across the head, so stimulating those lines can boost wellbeing and energy.

3 chin wipe and jaw circles

To increase metabolism, open up energy meridians and reduce tension, use alternating hands to wipe from the point of your chin to your collarbone. Repeat 12 times. Then relax your jaw, unclench your teeth and make deep friction circles into your jaw muscles.

4 mona lisa smile

This may sound surprising, but your facial expressions can actually alter how you feel. To lift your spirits, bring a slight smile to your lips. Smiling and breathing deeply, place your index fingers in the corners of your mouth and gently push them up. Release and repeat for 10–20 smiles, or until you begin to feel a Mona Lisa smile.

Pep Up at Work
- Revive your energy with an aromatherapy mister scented with rosemary or bergamot essential oils.
- Dry eyes make the rest of the body feel listless. Restore moisture to tired eyes by making gentle fingertip circles on your closed eyes.
- In Chinese medicine, the kidneys are considered an energy reservoir. Lean forwards and use your palms to gently rub your kidneys (located at the base of the ribs) and lower back.

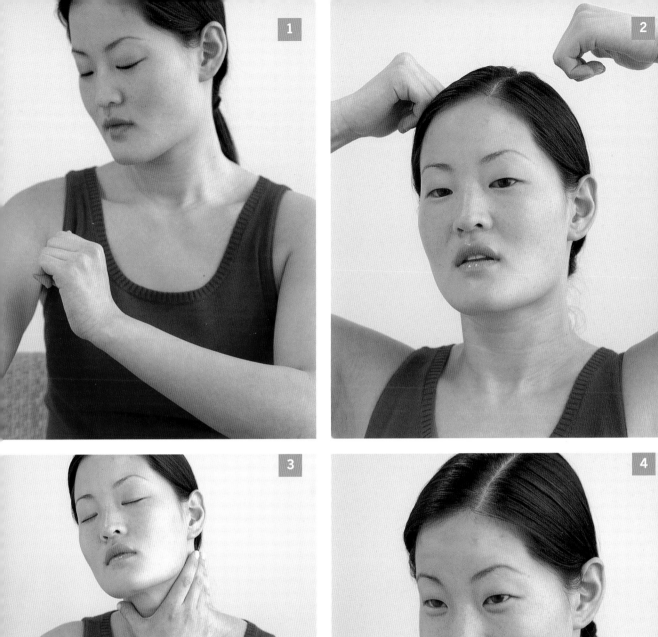

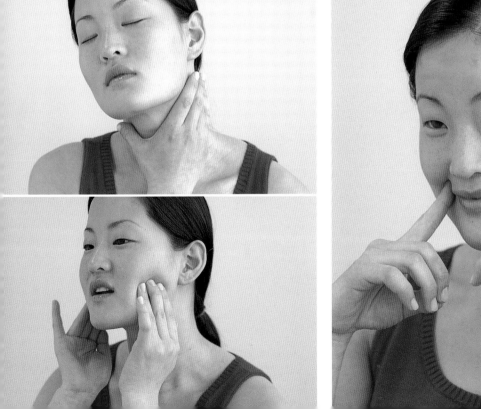

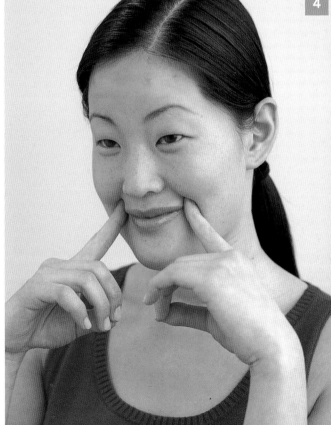

chill

Stress can be a killer – literally – but in our fast-paced society, it's worn like a badge of honour. Think about it, though: in the rat race, no one really wins. The key is to find a balance and make time to chill out. Touch is a subtle but potent stress-management tool that helps get you out of the race and back into your life.

key benefits

► Reduces stress

► Restores concentration

► Integrates calmness into your day

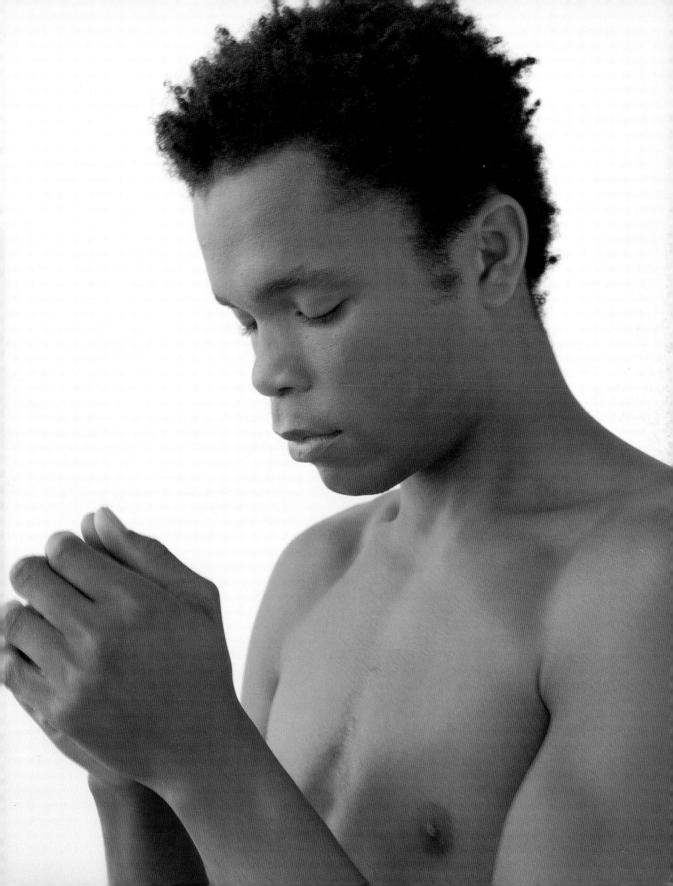

de-stress

Find a comfortable spot – for instance, a futon on the
floor makes a great base for this massage. Then ask
a friend to follow these steps and help melt away stress.

1 energy head hold and face strokes

Rub your hands together, then rest them behind your partner's ears
with your thumbs above. Imagine transferring warmth and energy
through your hands. Don't press; just hold the head lightly for a
minute or so. Next, use featherlight thumb and finger strokes across
the forehead, cheeks and jaw, drawing towards the ears. Trace the
lips, nose and ears delicately with your fingertips.

2 hand glide

Support your partner's hand comfortably between your hands. Hold
for three breaths. Then glide from his wrist to his fingertips, pressing
and pulling very gently. Repeat sequence three times on each hand.

3 foot circles and slides

To give a stress-relieving foot massage, press down firmly with your
thumb and circle across the entire bottom of your partner's foot.
Then slide your hand up the ankle into the calf muscles, squeezing
with your thumb and fingers. Ask your partner to tell you if the
pressure is too hard; avoid causing pain. Repeat on the other foot.

4 energy rock

To balance your partner's energy and help him relax (or fall asleep),
rest your right hand below his navel and your left hand on his
forehead. Then rock your right hand gently, using only enough
pressure to roll his hips. Do this for 20 seconds, then rest for 20
seconds. Keep going for a few minutes, until he sighs – or snores!

Soothing Scents

- When anxiety strikes, calm your
  spirit with a whiff of bergamot,
  jasmine, patchouli or rose essential
  oil dabbed onto a handkerchief.
- Pressing a cool flannel against
  your forehead can help you feel
  restored; soak the flannel in water
  mixed with 5 drops of essential oil.
- Or try an invigorating foot soak with
  5 drops of peppermint oil in a bowl
  of cold or hot water. To really relax,
  add 5–10 drops of soothing lavender
  or chamomile oil to a warm bath.
  Sink in and soak your cares away.

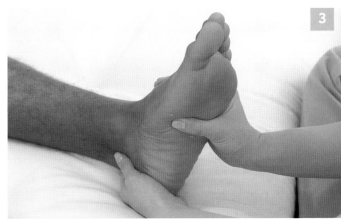

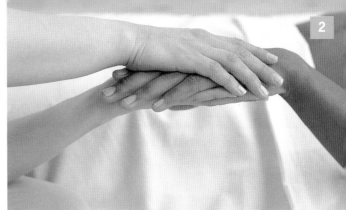

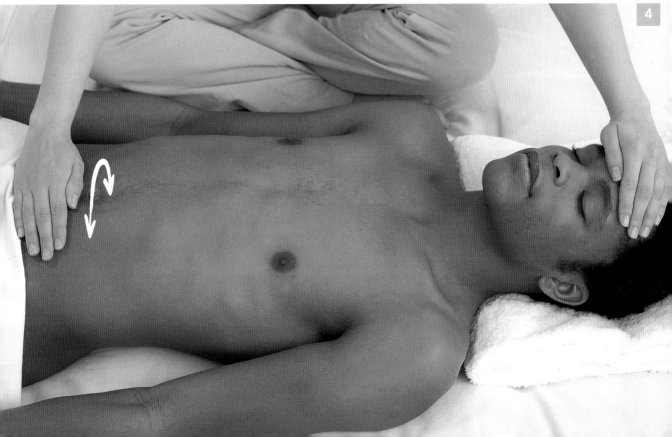

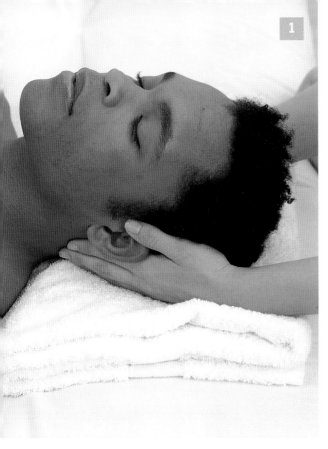

stealth-help

If you're stressed to the hilt and can't slip off for a massage, take the do-it-yourself route. Unwind and energise – and no one need know you're doing it. All you need is your own body (and maybe a golf ball).

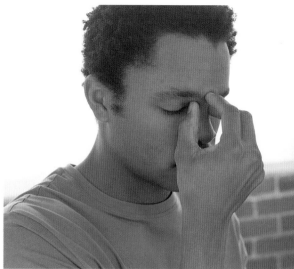

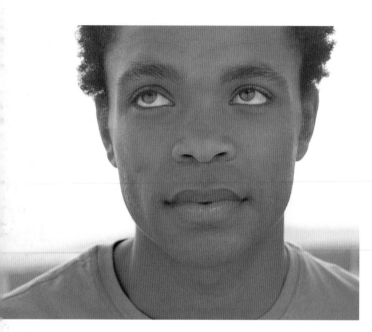

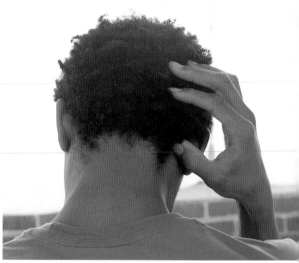

1 eye circles

Holding your eyes in one position for long periods fatigues the whole body. Ease eye tension by holding your head still and looking far up, down, right and left. Hold each position for a full breath. You can do this with your eyes open or closed, whichever you prefer.

2 nose pinches

To ease breathing and stimulate energy meridians, pinch the bridge of your nose repeatedly while taking three full breaths. Then rub the sides of your nose in small circles, working from bridge to tip.

3 neck nods

Press your right thumb into the base of your skull near your right ear and nod 3–6 times. Work your thumb across the ridge of your skull towards the spine, nodding at each spot. Repeat on left side.

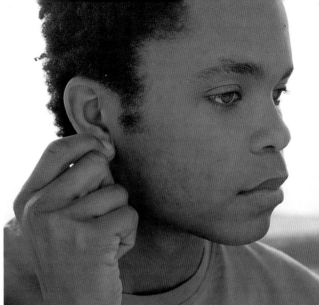

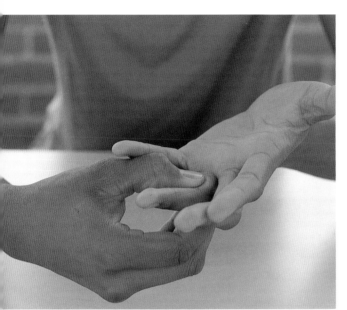

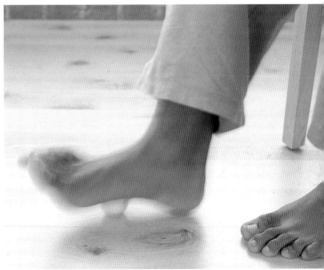

4 finger massage

According to Chinese medicine, massaging the fingers can help manage emotions. Give it a try by squeezing, rubbing or holding the pertinent area: the thumb for worry, index finger for depression, middle finger for impatience, ring finger for anger and little finger for fear.

5 ear rub

The ear has more than 100 reflexology points. Try massaging these points to relax specific body parts: the earlobes for the head, the middle part of the ear for the trunk, and the top for the lower body.

6 foot roll

For a fast foot massage, roll a foot over a golf ball. Stimulate reflexology points for the whole body by rolling the ball all along the bottom of each foot, then grip and squeeze the ball with your toes.

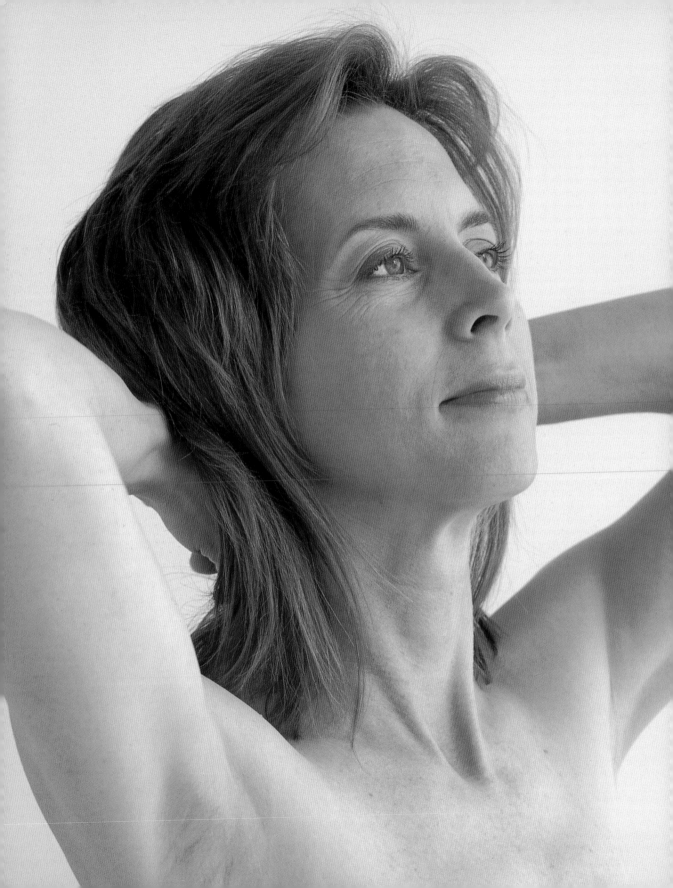

escape

Travel, whether for work or pleasure, can take a toll on our bodies, from the threat of blood clots caused by inactivity to the discomfort of jet lag. But you can soften your journey's impact with a little preparation and a few massage strokes. Wherever your destination, you'll arrive ready to hit the ground running.

key benefits

▶ Staves off travel tiredness and stiffness

▶ Keeps legs flexible

▶ Improves circulation and breathing

in-flight workout

Sitting for long periods may cause muscles to stiffen and impede blood circulation. Head off problems with stretches you can do discreetly in your aeroplane seat.

1 breathing rib stretch

Upper body stretches, combined with deep breathing, can improve oxygenation and combat listlessness and stiffness while you're travelling. Sit facing forwards in your seat. Reach across your chest with your right hand and grasp the armrest on the opposite side. Lean to the right, stretching your side for the count of five slow breaths. Then repeat this stretch on the other side.

2 chest stretch

To help get your circulation moving and open your chest for deeper breathing, press both elbows firmly back into your seat, arch your chest forwards and breathe deeply three times while maintaining the arm pressure. Relax, rounding your back. Repeat three to five times.

3 leg compression and foot alphabet

Improve leg circulation by using the sports massage technique of compression. Cross one leg over the other and firmly press the heel of your hand into your calf with rhythmic, pumping strokes, working the muscles from ankle to knee. Then increase blood flow to your leg by "drawing" the letters of the alphabet with your big toe. Switch legs and repeat the sequence with the other leg.

4 thigh compression

Bracing your left arm with your right and using the flat of your fist against your leg, firmly press down, then release, along the muscles on the top of your thigh, rhythmically rocking your weight forwards and back. Start above your knee, press in and lift up, moving a centimetre at a time towards your hip. Switch sides and repeat on the other leg.

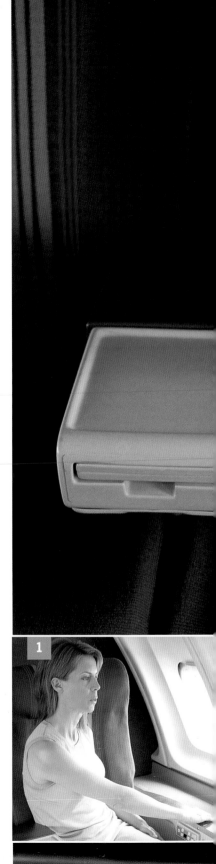

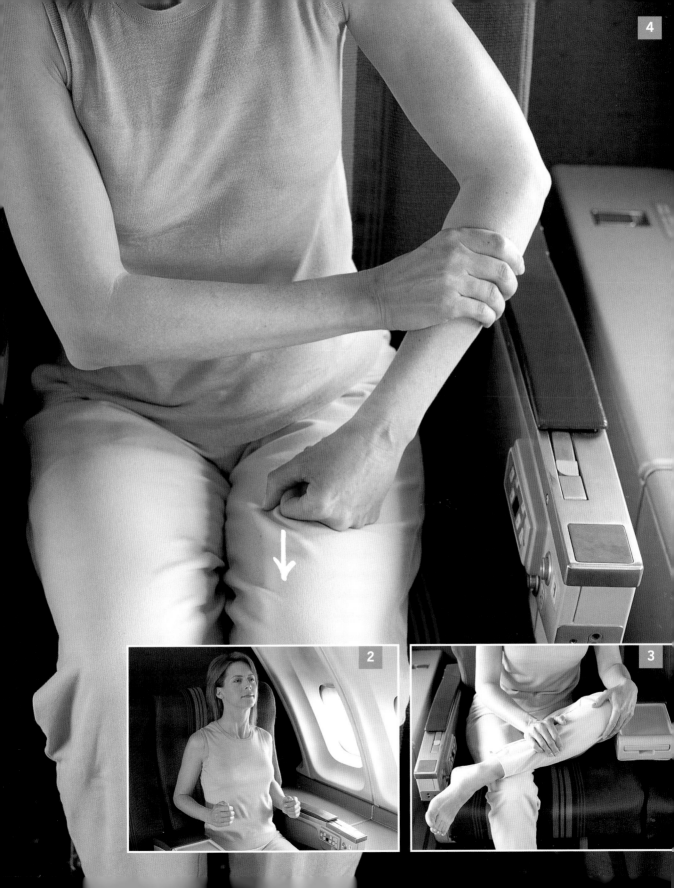

bon voyage

Have a friend lend a hand with these steps to zap travellers' woes like headaches from stuffy planes and the stiffness caused by carting luggage. Then return the favour, so you both can enjoy your trip to its fullest.

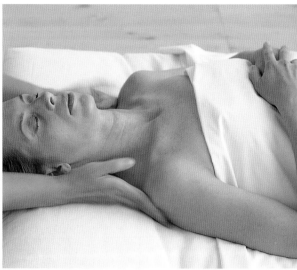

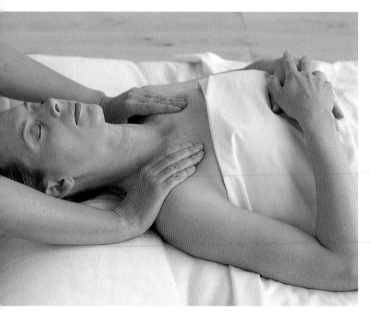

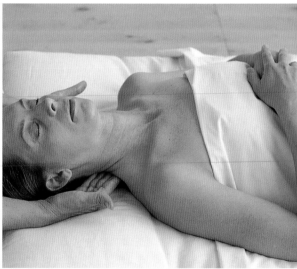

1 chest sweep

Sitting or kneeling behind your partner, warm a small amount of massage oil in your hands, rest your palms on her shoulders, press the flats of your fingers into the chest muscles and push your hands out towards her arms. Take care not to press down on the collarbones. Complete the sequence with a shoulder press followed by neck sweeps and circles (steps 2–3).

2 shoulder press

Next, sweep your fingers around the outside of her shoulders, then swing them underneath, pressing firmly into the muscles with your fingertips, and pull your hands in towards the base of her neck.

3 neck sweeps and circles

Press into the muscles at the base of her neck along either side of the spine; lean back and stroke towards her skull. Using fingertips, circle into the skull's base from the spine outwards. Repeat steps 1–3 five times.

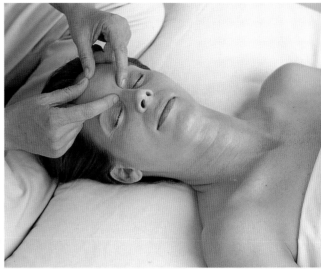

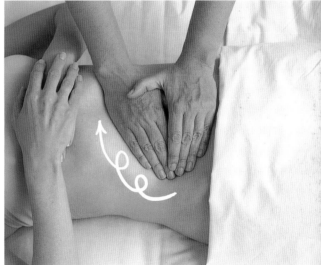

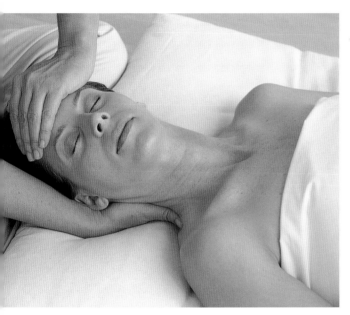

4 headache energy hold

With your right hand, lightly hold your fingers
and thumb on either side of your partner's spine
at the base of her neck. Rest your left hand gently
on her forehead and hold while she takes ten
deep breaths. Finish by stroking her forehead
with light wiping motions up and back.

5 sinus point press

Press your index fingers lightly into the bone
indentations above the bridge of her nose. Gently
vibrate your fingertips as she takes three full breaths.
Repeat at the outside bottom edge of the nostrils.

6 abdomen circles

Very gently press in between her navel and right
hip. Use small clockwise circles to move towards the
right ribs. Staying just below the ribs, circle across
to her left ribs, then down to the left hip.

excel

You want to play hard, perform at your peak and avoid injury. Sports massage techniques get you pumped up and ready, then help undo damage at the day's end. Sports strokes ease pain, speed circulation and separate stuck muscle fibres that can impair speed, strength and endurance. So get out there and give it all you've got.

key benefits

▶ Warms you up or cools you down

▶ Improves performance and power

▶ Helps prevent injury

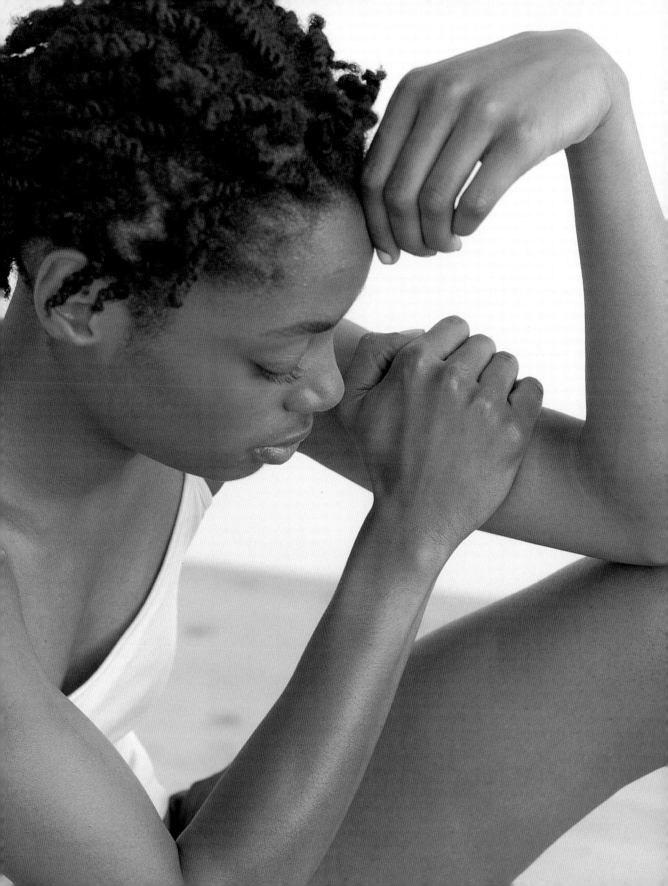

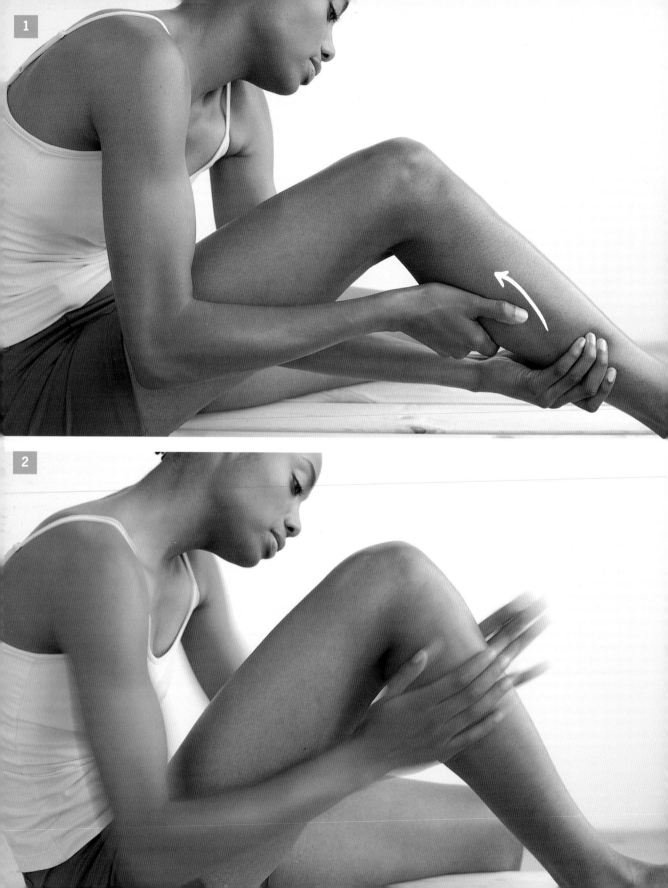

work it out

Massage is great before, during or after a workout. To loosen up your leg muscles, do all the strokes below on one leg, then perform the same routine on the other leg.

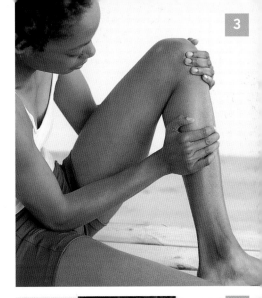

1 calf glide

To flush fluids up towards the heart, make a tight seal with the edge of your index fingers and thumbs, and alternately pull each hand up your calf, from your ankle to your knee, ten times.

2 calf roll

Press your palms firmly into the back of your calf, and rapidly push up with one hand while simultaneously pulling down with the other, creating a rolling motion. Roll your calf for about 30 seconds.

3 calf compression

Relieve fluid congestion and soreness by rhythmically pumping your calf. Press the heel of your palm in towards the bone, release and repeat the compression ten times, moving from ankle to knee.

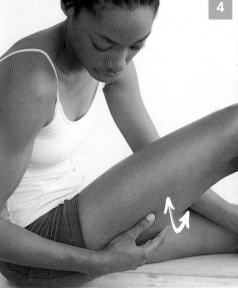

4 hamstrings jostle

Tight hamstrings slow you down, decrease leg power and wear you out more quickly. Relax tension in your hamstrings by grasping the muscles on the underside of your thigh and waggling them loosely from side to side. Jostle these muscles, moving up and down the length of your thigh, switching to the other hand if one tires.

5 thigh compression

Squeeze out painful lactic acid and metabolic wastes by compressing your quadriceps (on the tops of your thighs). With the heels of both palms, press into your thigh muscles, squeezing towards the bone in a pumping action. Release the pressure and move to a new spot, repeating from knee to hip. For extra power as you perform this motion, rock forwards as you press in and lean back on your release.

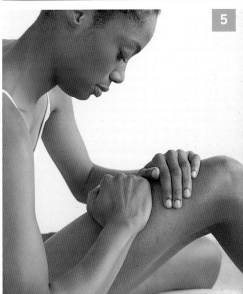

well armed

Improve circulation with compression strokes, then use pressure and cross-fibre friction to release painful muscle spasms and free up tissue around muscles for peak performance. Be sure to work both arms.

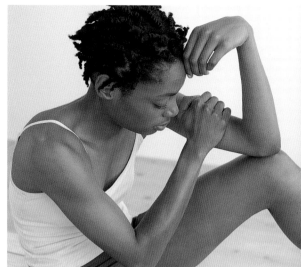

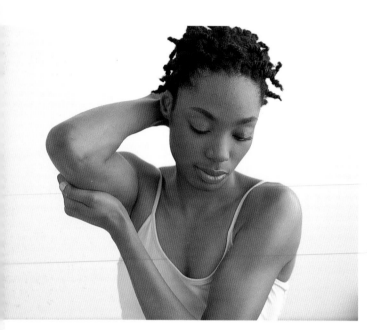

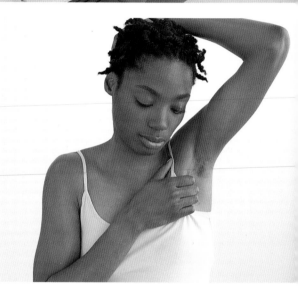

1 triceps compression

To flush out painful metabolic wastes, squeeze the heel of your hand and your fingers together on the triceps muscle on the underside of your arm. Release. Repeat, starting at your elbow and moving a little at a time towards your armpit.

2 biceps compression

With your palm against the inside of your biceps and fingers wrapped around to the back, squeeze the heel of the palm and fingers towards each other.

3 armpit squeeze

With one hand braced on the back of your head, sink your fingertips into the front edge of your armpit, getting under your chest muscles. Squeeze your thumb and fingers together. Work the length of the muscle from top to bottom.

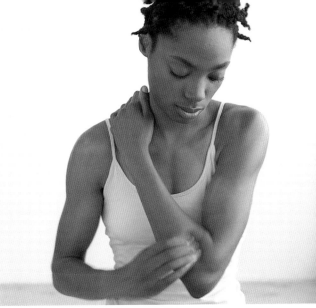

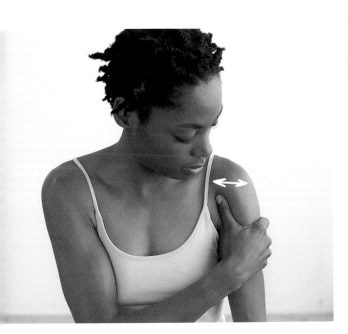

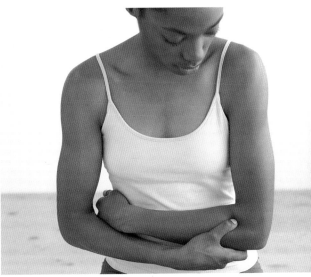

4 upper arm cross-fibre rub

The front of your arm has ropy muscles that can get tight. Move across the grain of them with your thumb using cross-fibre friction, starting from just below your collarbone and working down to the inside of your elbow. (See page 17 ◄ for more about cross-fibre friction.)

5 forearm cross-fibre rub

Sink your fingers into the muscles on the top of your forearm and rub across them, feeling the muscles roll under the pressure. Release your grip slightly, reposition and repeat from elbow to wrist.

6 sore spot presses

Gently probe your arms for tender spots. When you find one, breathe in and press your thumb into it as you exhale; hold for 10–30 seconds while breathing normally. Release gradually. Repeat three times.

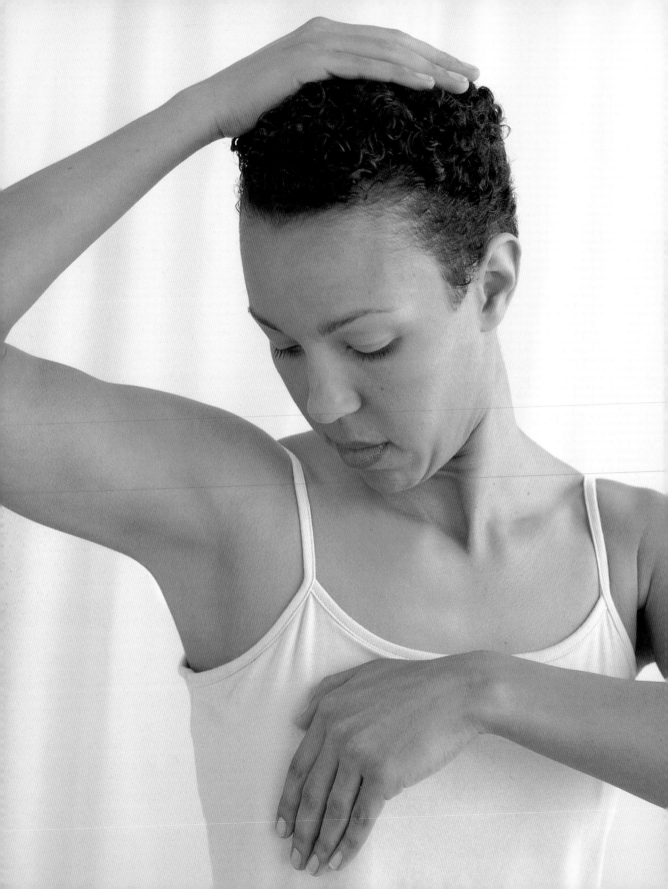

comfort

The menstrual cycle can literally be a pain, yet it is an inevitable – and natural – part of women's lives. Touch is a potent tool to connect with your body during its most sensitive time of the month, helping to stroke away discomfort and swelling. Both cramps and premenstrual symptoms can be soothed with massage.

key benefits

▶ Reduces cyclical swelling

▶ Helps alleviate PMS symptoms

▶ Lessens menstrual pain

put yourself at ease

Find a place that's quiet and private and try these simple and effective treatments aimed at lessening cyclical discomfort in your breasts, back and belly.

1 breast lymphatic sweeps

Relieve the pain of swollen breasts with a series of gentle gliding strokes. Using the side of your index finger to exert light pressure, make six sweeps from the centre of a breast out into four directions: to your armpit, then up to the collarbone, then to the breastbone and finally downwards. Repeat on the other breast.

2 knee circles

Knee circles can often help relieve lower back pain. With your back flat on the floor, bring your knees towards your chest and slowly circle them, gently pulling your knees across your abdomen from the right side to the left and back. Circle your legs ten times.

3 lower back stretch

Kneel, sit back on your heels and rest your arms on the floor with palms up. Place your head on the floor and breathe deeply into your lower back for five breaths or until pain subsides.

4 waist bend and energy hold

To help ease abdominal pain, touch the soles of your feet together, grasp them with both hands (but don't pull upwards), inhale fully and lean slowly forwards on an exhale. Round your back and gently aim your forehead towards your feet, but make sure you only go as far as feels comfortable. Hold for 3–5 deep breaths.

Finish with an energy hold. Lie flat on the floor. Rub your hands together vigorously until they're warm and then lay them on your abdomen, with your right hand below your navel and your left hand above it. Using your hands, gently rock your torso from side to side for about 20 seconds. Be still for 20 seconds, visualising your hands' warmth easing your pain. Repeat, alternating rocking and stillness.

Scent Saviours

• Aromatherapy can help relieve many problems during a menstrual cycle. To aid with depression or mood swings, add 3 drops of bergamot, jasmine, lavender or sandalwood essential oil to water and use with scented sprays or vaporisers.

• To help relieve fluid retention, add 5 drops of patchouli or rosemary essential oil to 2 teaspoons of massage oil and pour it in bathwater or use it to massage your abdomen.

• Cramps can be relieved with cool compresses. Add 2–3 drops of clary sage or 5 drops of chamomile essential oil to a bowl of cold water, dip in a towel, wring it out and place it on the abdomen.

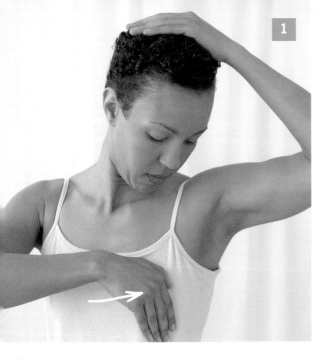

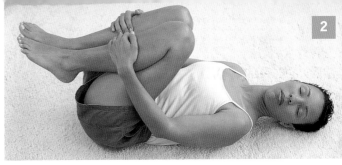

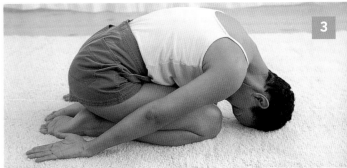

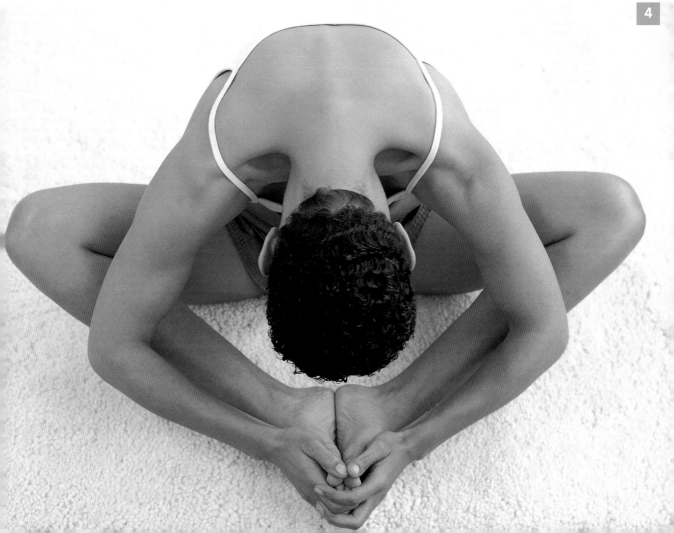

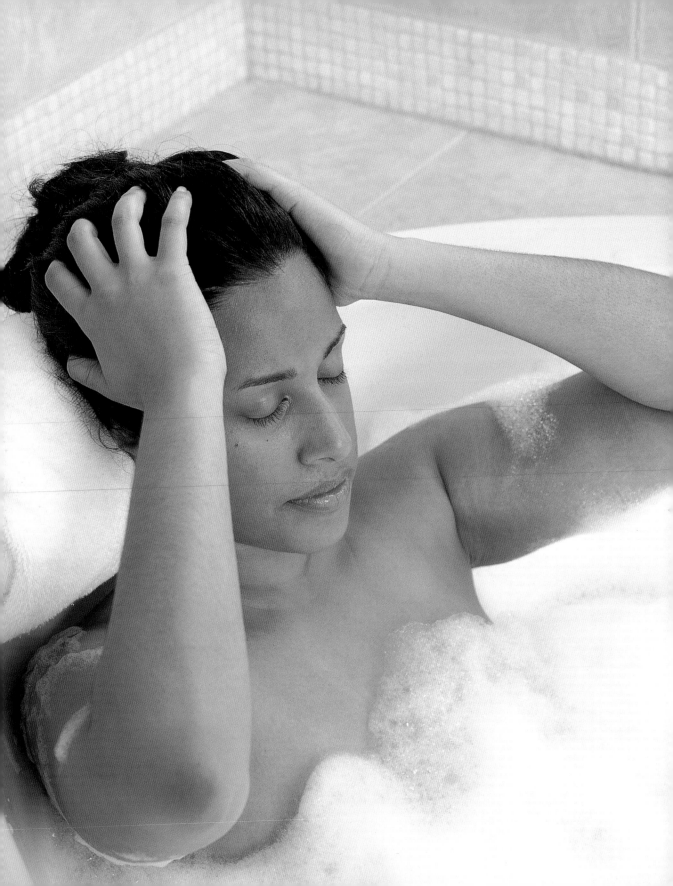

retreat

You've seized the day and squeezed it dry. Now it's time to let go. A hot bath is ideal for softening life's sharp edges and easing tense muscles. Melt into the bath, revel in steam sweetened with exotic aromas and wash away the day's cares. While you're soaking, indulge yourself with some soothing self-massage techniques.

key benefits

► Helps you forget your worries

► Releases the day's tension

► Helps you unwind before bedtime

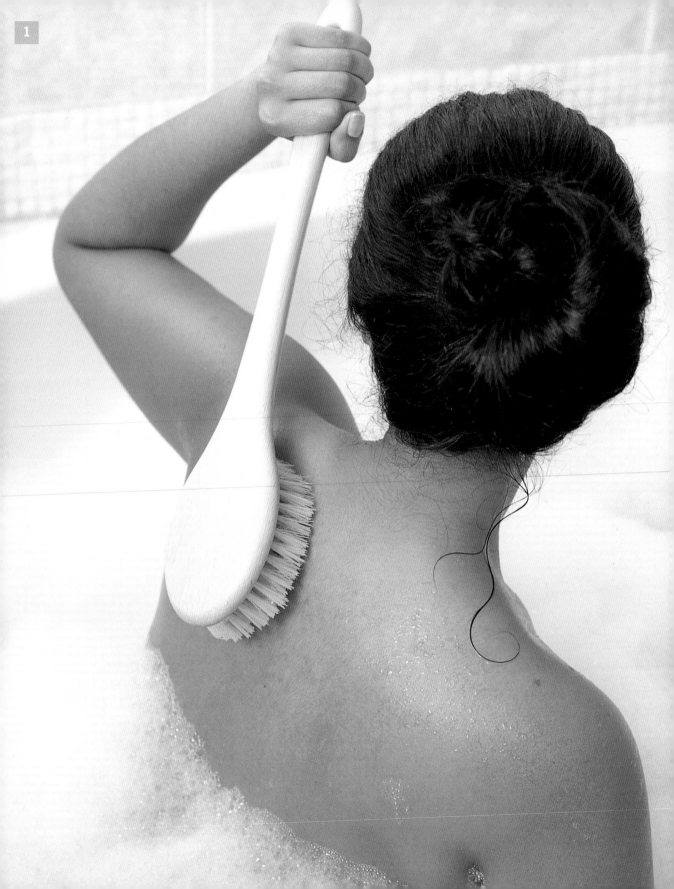

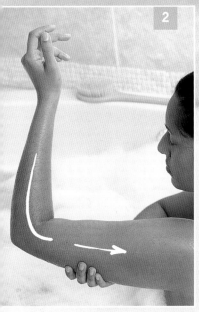

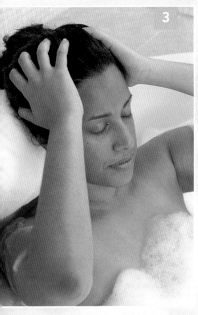

undo the day

For a relaxing evening, gather your favourite bathing supplies and aromatherapy essential oils and sink into the bath for some soothing, sleep-inspiring moves.

1 back brush

Dry (or wet) brushing your skin is one of the best ways to move toxins through the superficial lymphatic system just below the skin's surface. Brush up and down your back using light pressure, covering where you can comfortably reach. Then brush your arms and legs, but brush only with an upward motion (in lymphatic work, always move fluids towards your heart).

2 arm glides

To soothe overworked arms, turn one hand palm-side up. Wrap the fingers of your other hand around it at the wrist and glide with firm pressure from wrist to elbow to underarm. Repeat several times with increasing pressure; repeat on the other arm.

3 scalp scrub

Wash that day right out of your hair by rubbing and scrubbing your scalp. Make firm circles with your fingertips, using your nails for extra stimulation to help relax tight scalp muscles and stimulate energy meridians. (A scalp scrub helps ease tension even without shampoo – so you can try this on dry land, too.)

To add aromatherapy benefits to your bath time, add to the bath water a tablespoon of bath or massage oil and 5–15 drops of your favourite essential oil. Sandalwood is said to sedate, soothe depression and ease tension; ylang-ylang to relax, ease anxiety and relieve insomnia; jasmine to lift your mood (and act as an aphrodisiac); lavender to balance moods and soothe frayed nerves; rose to inspire romance and lift your spirits; and patchouli to leave you feeling uplifted, earthy and sensual.

dream

In healing slumber, the dust of each day settles, the body repairs itself and dreams clear the mind. If deep sleep is elusive and you're tired of dragging through your days, enlist the calming effects of touch. Alone or with a partner, you can quieten your mind and welcome peaceful slumber with a caress.

key benefits

- ▶ Helps ensure a good night's sleep
- ▶ Soothes your body and soul
- ▶ Helps you relinquish worries

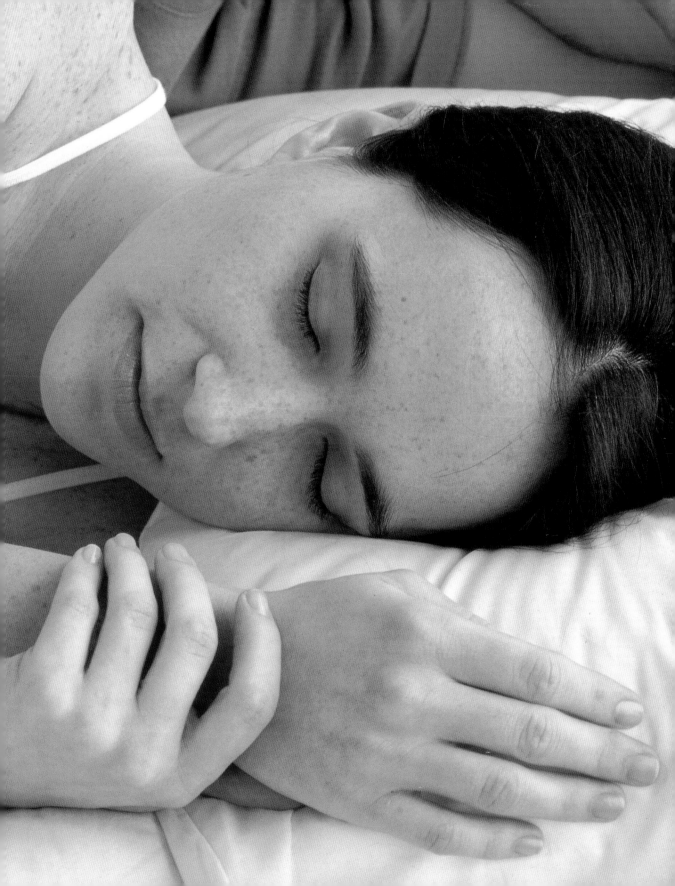

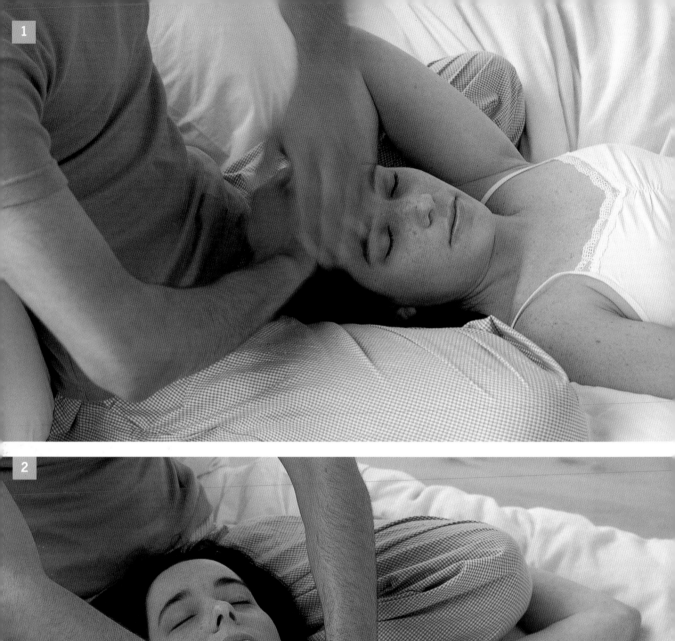

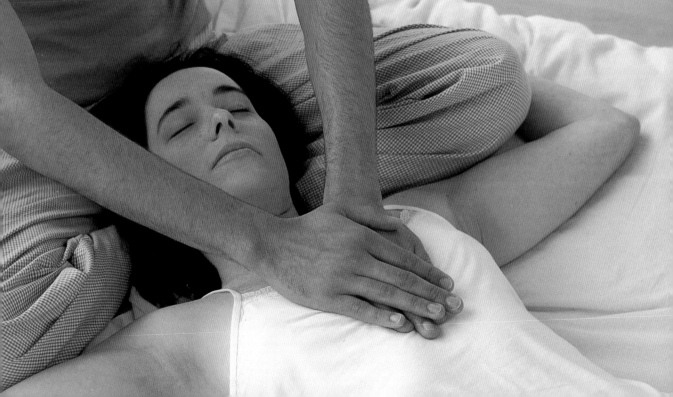

sweet dreams

A partner's gentle touch at bedtime can work wonders. These simple steps will leave you feeling comforted and cherished – and ready to sleep like a baby.

1 forehead stroking

The simple act of stroking back the hair has soothed millions of children to sleep for centuries. Eastern massage practitioners believe this is because it releases a built-up density of energy around the head. (Besides, it feels wonderful!) Lightly stroke your partner's forehead upwards, brushing back her hair with alternating hands.

2 heart hold

Make use of what healers worldwide know: sending love through your hands is powerful medicine. Rest both hands on your partner's heart and feel her breath rise and fall for five breaths.

3 arm sway

Simple, gentle swaying can be profoundly relaxing. Gentle swinging creates awareness of where tensions are held and encourages release. Hold your partner's hand comfortably, and lift and swing her arm from side to side. Vary your speed and her arm angles to encourage letting go, and sway for a minute or so. Repeat with her other arm.

4 back scratch

A good back scratching is also soothing. Superficial nerves on the skin's surface savour stimulation (even at bedtime). Scratch all over her back, applying soft or moderate pressure, whichever she prefers.

5 cradle rock

Snuggle up behind your partner, rest one hand on her abdomen between her navel and ribs, and gently rock your bodies back and forth. This position not only feels comforting, it also helps create a deep and peaceful sense of connection between the two of you.

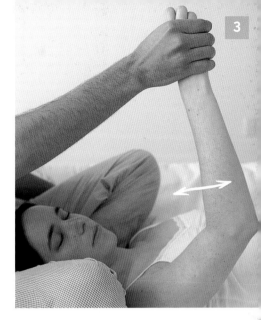

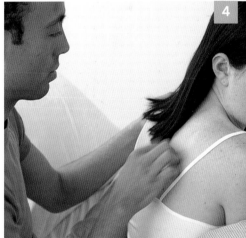

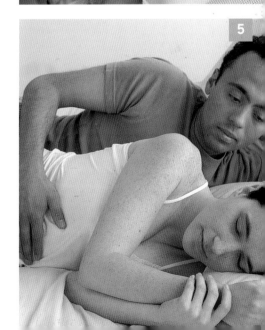

rest easy

Knock yourself out: if you're feeling too keyed up to sleep, use these basic tips to still soul and body at bedtime. (If you're experiencing chronic insomnia, it would be wise to seek professional help.)

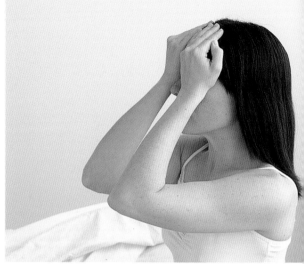

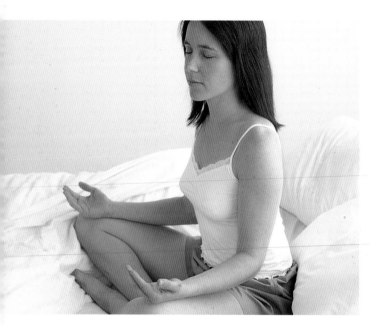

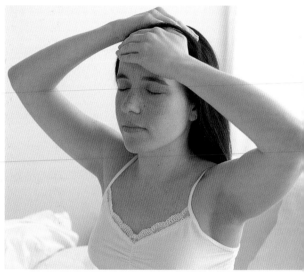

1 stillness position

Help quieten mind and body by sitting in this classic meditation position and reviewing your day's experiences. Let thoughts stream through your mind for a few minutes. Study them; then let them go, allowing your mind to clear.

2 eye cupping

We don't often think of it, but our busy eyes do carry tension. Rub your hands together until warm, then gently mould the heels of your hands to your closed eyes. Breathe deeply and repeat.

3 forehead stroking

Soothing forehead strokes help release built-up energy around your head. With closed eyes, start at your eyebrows and alternately sweep each hand 10–15 times up your forehead and into your hair.

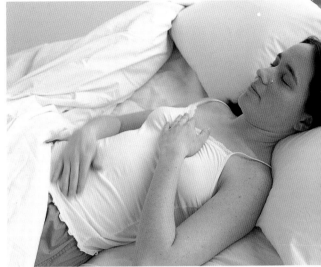

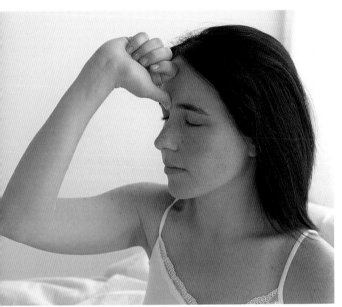

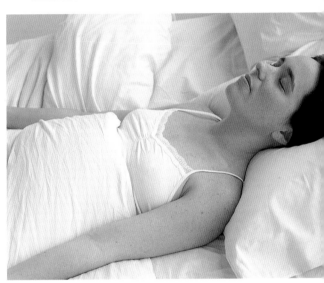

4 point press

Press lightly into the acupressure point between your eyebrows at the bridge of the nose to relax and calm your central nervous system. Hold the point for three full, deep breaths, relaxing and letting go of stressful thoughts.

5 belly breathing

Breathing deeply can induce a restful state. Lying with knees bent, rest your right hand on your belly, left hand on your chest. Breathe in and out fully, so that your belly expands more than your chest.

6 corpse pose

Lie in this relaxing yoga pose: legs straight out and slightly apart, toes pointed outwards and arms beside, but not touching, your body. Turn your palms up, close your eyes and focus on your breath.

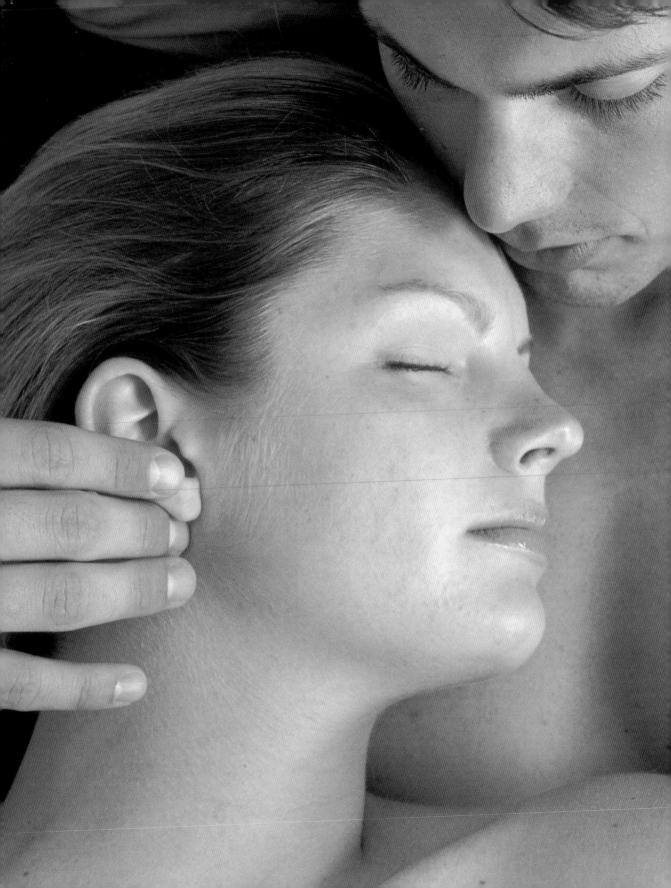

seduce

When passion's flames are ready to be lit, sensual massage can spark desire. Explore, arouse, tempt. Touch like new lovers. Trace secret paths, feeling your partner's heart quicken and pulse race. Stroke each other with passionate purpose, with love and lust lashed together. Be bold and try something new.

key benefits

- ▶ Stimulates erogenous zones
- ▶ Enhances intimacy
- ▶ Gets you in the mood for love

make some moves

Sensual massage uses light strokes on sensitive zones. Find a comfortable, private space, tune into your partner and explore. Go ahead, turn up the heat.

1 belly and breastbone trace

Starting just below your partner's navel, slowly trace your fingertips across her lower belly and along the top of her hip-bones. Trace inwards at her waist to her navel; circle it a few times. Glide up to the top of her breastbone. Slide outwards to her shoulders and breasts.

2 wrist strokes

Use featherlight strokes to brush your partner's wrist with fingertips and nails, moving across her palm and up each finger to the tip. Outline the sides of each finger, then retrace back to her wrist.

3 face trace

Stroke outwards along your partner's forehead. Begin between her brows and circle in along her cheekbones and up to the bridge of her nose. Slip your fingers down to her lips; outline and explore.

4 arm sweeps

Stroke the soft, sensitive skin of your partner's inner arms, elbows and forearms with light, easy sweeps of your hands. Use featherlight fingertip or nail strokes, lingering to circle the sensitive spots.

Amorous Aromas

Try mixing sensual touch with the stimulating effects of aromatherapy:

- Slip a tissue dabbed with a few drops of patchouli into your robe.
- Mist bed linens with rose spray, or add a few drops of jasmine to the rinse cycle when washing them.
- Tuck a cotton ball touched with ylang-ylang into a pillowcase.
- Add 5 drops of neroli to a small bowl of water and place it on the radiator for an alluring humidifier.
- Light aromatherapy candles – the ultimate mood-makers.

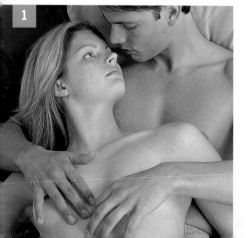

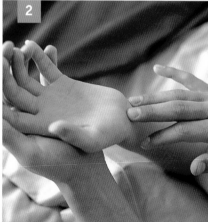

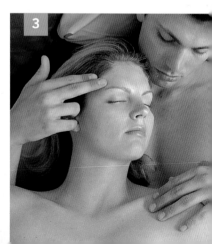

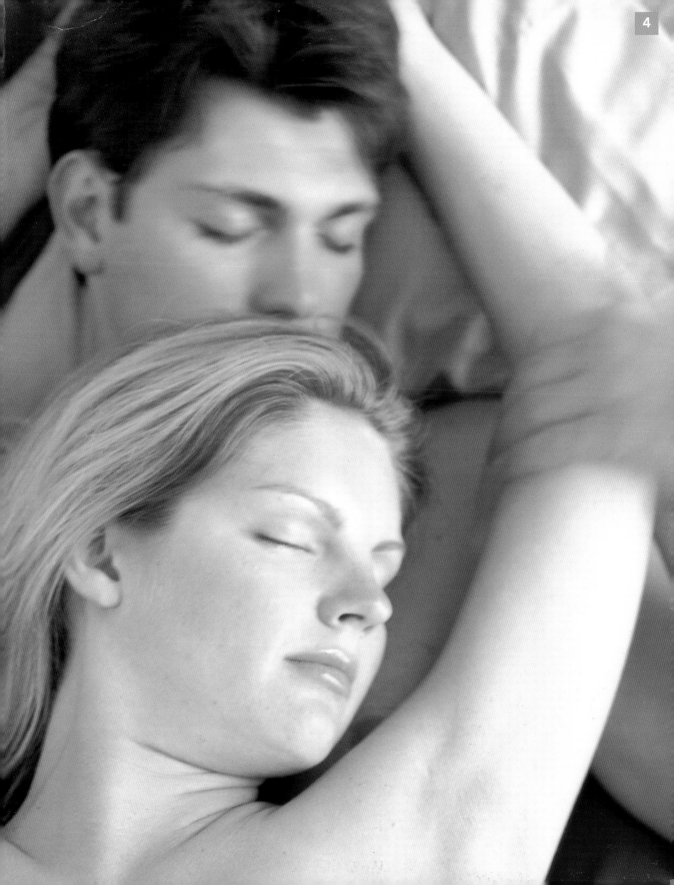

explore more

Now that you're both warmed up, try these tender stroking techniques to help unleash the sensualist in you and in your loving partner. The power of touch can further tantalise the two of you in fun new ways.

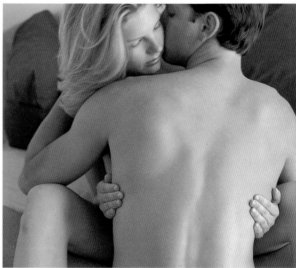

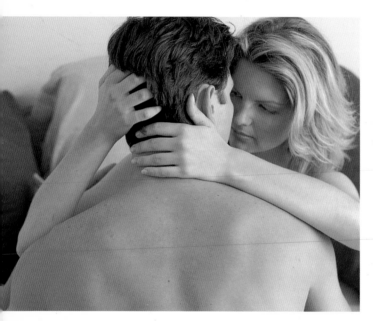

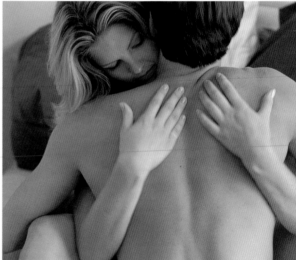

1 scalp strokes

With your fingernails, lightly scratch all over your partner's scalp, experimenting with pressure and moves. Delight him with small, delicate circles, then alternate with gentle, 2.5 cm-long raking strokes. Pay close attention to what he likes, then do it some more.

2 side strokes

Slide your hands up and down the contours of your partner's sides. Starting at his hip-bone, stroke up his hips, waist and ribs, and along the back of his arms and underarms. Be careful of ticklishness.

3 back strokes

Bewitch your partner with a variety of strokes, from delicate fingernail scratching to sensuous sweeping glides. Using long, smooth strokes, slide up and down his back between his neck and buttocks.

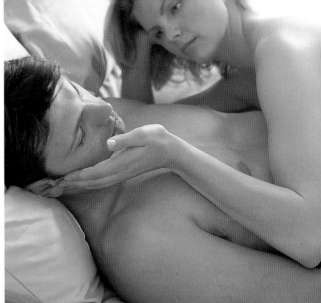

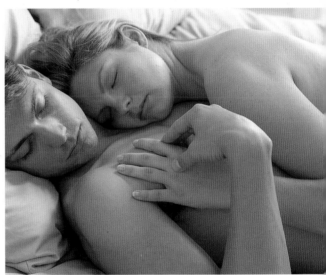

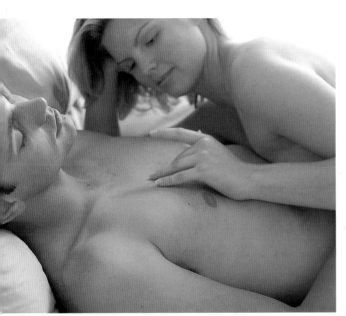

4 chest caress

Lying atop your partner, rest your hand in the middle of his chest, and breathe in sync, feeling his heartbeat. Then stroke his chest and belly, traversing their curves with your fingertips or nails, discovering sensual spots to explore further. Let your imagination run wild.

5 neck and face caress

Tantalise your lover with gentle strokes on his neck and face. With your fingertips, caress his throat from collarbone to chin; then glide up to his cheekbones and trace his ears. Very gently repeat these strokes using the backs of your fingernails.

6 full body caress

Slide along his body and breathe in unison, focusing on tactile sensations and the bond growing between you. Let your hands caress and explore.

index

acknowledgements

We wish to thank the following for their generous assistance with this book: additional photography by John Robbins, front cover, pages 6 (bottom left corner), 10, 12, 13, 52, front inside cover flap (centre and bottom), back inside cover flap (centre and bottom), back cover (top and centre); Joanna Brown, Jane Burley and Tracey Edwards from The Body Shop International; Peter Cieply, managing editor, and Susan Koenig, consulting editor, for the hardback edition; Lisa Milestone and Jackie Mancuso for design assistance; Gail Nelson-Bonebrake and Kate Washington for copyediting; Tom Hassett, Cynthia Rubin and Renée Myers for proofreading; Ken DellaPenta for indexing; Virginia McLean for research; make-up artist Christine Lucignano/Koko Represents; photo assistants Jessica Giblin, April Keener and Doug Muise; models David Andrade, Carla Caballero, Xavier Castellanos, Josh Ceazan, Samuel Celestine, Rebecca Chang, Margaret Cobbs, Sarah Coleman, Michele Crim, Joey Deleo, Ivola Demange, Jennifer "Lexi" Durst, Michelle Gagnon, Jessie Geevarghese, Devon Gill, Rebecca Handler, Todd Maderis, Jared Meyer, Lulu Monti, Ryan Mortensen, Mia Parler, Carmen Peirano, Patricia Quesada, Ellen Rhee, Monica Roseberry, Rachel Ruperto, Michael Schindele, Bridget Sullivan, Cynthia R. Wren, Crystal Wright and Lake Ziwa-Rodriguez; Erin Quon for lending photography locations.